The Eating Game

The simple truth to health and fat loss in the modern world

by

Dr. Shannon Paul Alexander D.C.

authorHOUSE

1663 LIBERTY DRIVE, SUITE 200
BLOOMINGTON, INDIANA 47403
(800) 839-8640
www.authorhouse.com

First published by AuthorHouse 11/23/04

ISBN: 1-4184-9224-8 (e)
ISBN: 1-4184-3161-3 (sc)

Library of Congress Control Number: 2004098768

Printed in the United States of America
Bloomington, Indiana

This book is printed on acid-free paper.

THE EATING GAME

The Eating Game is a to-the-point guide that explains the changes in our food supply and how they are affecting us, especially our efforts to lose weight. More and more people are experiencing health and weight problems as a result of our altered food supply. It has been my experience that while most people are concerned about their health, the majority are only willing to spend a small amount of time on the process of doing something about it.

The book is short by design and is aimed at beginners. I wanted to write a book that people could read quickly so they can get started right away. *The Eating Game* gives the reader the big picture in a simple format, of the changes in our food supply, and the science behind human health and fat loss. This is followed by a simple and effective solution that can be done by anyone.

The appendix contains a complete vitamin and mineral reference, a hypoallergenic food reference, and an explanation of food allergies and autoimmune diseases. These were placed at the back to avoid breaking the easy flow of the book and to provide a ready reference.

Shannon Paul Alexander D.C.

Dedicated to my son Zachary for making my world a better place, and to my family and friends for their undying support.

Thanks for Everything

TABLE OF CONTENTS

"Man's mind, once stretched by a new idea, never regains its original dimensions."

-Oliver Wendel Holmes

INTRODUCTION

This book is as much about your mind as it is about diet and exercise. To a large extent, our daily habits have determined whether we're fat or thin, healthy or diseased. One day at the gym will not get you into shape any more than one cigarette will give you cancer. It's the culmination of hundreds, if not thousands, of days that will decide your fate. I know that if I can change the way you think about what you do each day, you will begin to change your habits, which will change the way you feel and, eventually, the way you look "for as a man thinks, so he shall become."

You will see that just about every disorder you can suffer from has a nutritional component that involves mistakes you probably make on a daily basis. The most outward sign of this disease process is excessive bodyfat, a problem that is now epidemic in America.

I have spent years sifting through the hype and hoopla of diets and nutrition searching for the least common denominator between health and nutrition. It turns out that there is one (actually over sixty that function as one). It is a simple concept that will be abundantly clear by the end of this book. You need all the nutrients you are about to read about each day. We already apply this logic to our pets. The more the perceived value of the animal, such as a racehorse or a show dog, the more that is invested in proper nutrition. Everyone knows that if you want a fat, unhealthy dog all you have to do is feed him what you're eating. It is a shame that we sometimes fail to recognize the great value in ourselves.

The evidence is overwhelming that most of the essential nutrients we need to remain healthy have been stripped from our food. Not acknowledging this is the reason degenerative diseases are on the rise and why we are getting fatter. I'll examine evidence that will change the way you think about the food you've been eating. Then I'll show you exactly what you can do about it.

I have tried to make this book as short as possible because I know that confusion, more often than laziness, keeps people from taking action. Still, I am only able to cover a fraction of the mountain of evidence showing that we have depleted our farmlands, degraded our food, contaminated our water, and polluted our air. And the enormous benefits to be gained through proper nutritional supplementation and simple lifestyle changes.

This book was written for you because you are living right now. Whether you know it or not, you are involved in a game between your money and your health. You're up against the food industry, pharmaceutical companies, the diet industry, and even the government. For them, the prize is profit, and they know you and your biology well. They know how to play their game. Do you? When you consider that you have no choice but to play and the stakes are high, you might as well play to win. Your very life may depend on it.

It makes no difference if you are an athlete or a couch potato, this information applies to you, so use it to your advantage. I will show you where to start and why. The rest will be up to you. If you are willing to spend thirty seconds a day to turn on your blender, you'll be well on your way to winning this game. The program is so easy anyone can use it to undo a multitude of ills. You just have to take that first step. It's one you'll never regret taking.

Once you begin there's no hurry, your body responds to what you do most often over time, so use the program to get started today. Remember that fitness is a personal journey, not a destination. You can't store it. Your health depends on what you did yesterday, not six months ago. Each of us must learn to care for our own bodies, since we alone live in it, and we alone will bear the consequences of eating habits and a lifestyle out of balance with our natural biological requirements.

"Knowing others is wisdom, knowing yourself is Enlightenment."

-LAO-TZU

CHAPTER 1 – YOU ARE NOT ALONE

Today, widespread nutritional deficiencies are so common that just about everyone can consider themselves affected-and that means you! It's a universal problem that's been approached with so much misguided advice from our doctors, the government, and the nutritional industry; it's no wonder nothing is improving.

Let us begin by taking a realistic look at what you're up against. In 1988, *the Surgeon General reported that more than two thirds of all deaths in the United States involve nutrition.* Heart disease, cancer, and diabetes alone will kill two out of three Americans. The percentage of overweight adults in the U.S. has doubled since 1991; today, nearly 60% are overweight. The rate of obesity has increased by over 50% in the last forty years. Arthritis, allergies, fatigue, impotence, depression, Alzheimer's, osteoporosis, kidney disease and many other degenerative disorders are also on a dramatic rise. You may be surprised to learn that these are all different manifestations of the same disease – poor nutrition.

So, what are you going to do about it? Statistically, you will do absolutely nothing. You will follow your overweight American brethren like lemmings over a cliff. You may ask some questions along the way, or even dabble with leaving the pack, but only about five percent will succeed.

What about the diet and exercise craze that's supposedly sweeping America, all those before and after pictures? It's just marketing. All commercial diet programs even the medically supervised ones have an over 95% failure rate. The people who take them either drop out or gain back all the lost weight.

Research shows that we're actually eating more. According to the Department of Agriculture, per capita consumption of food has increased 8% from 1990 to 2000. That translates into an extra 140 pounds of food a year per person.

If you were to check the records of Americas health clubs you'd find that the average member shows up less than one time per week. In fact, less than 10% of adults aged 18-65 do any regular exercise at all (20 minutes or more three times a week).

Will a miracle drug come along to solve your problems? Don't get your hopes up, drugs are toxic and pharmaceutical companies are big business. We've come to rely on chemicals and technology to treat the symptoms caused by nutritional deficiencies. Most of these treatments don't cure anything. They merely mask one problem and cause a new one with their side effects. Drugs for cholesterol, depression, impotence, weight loss, the list goes on and on, even our children are routinely medicated.

There are advertisements that recommend taking an aspirin a day to help prevent a heart attack. They fail to mention that even a single aspirin can leave your digestive tract bleeding. Heart attacks are not caused by an aspirin deficiency. We've been sold weight loss drugs that were so toxic they caused irreversible heart damage in just months. The overuse of antibiotics has lead to drug resistant bacteria and weakened immune systems. Even breast cancer prevention campaigns recommend yearly mammograms, a procedure that exposes breast tissue to radiation. Radiation causes cancer, and though many of these types of procedures have their uses, this is not preventative medicine.

Our health care system is rooted in the study of disease instead of the study of health, because that's where the money is. What we really have is a *sick care system,* and you don't want to be part of it. Crackpot potions, diets, and drugs are everywhere, most of them don't live up to their billing, and may even harm you because they are out of line with your evolutionary requirements. Don't spend another dime on them until you know what you're doing.

"The most beautiful thing we can experience is the mysterious.
It is the source of all true art and science."

- Albert Einstein 1930

CHAPTER 2 - YOUR BODY – A MIRACLE OF NATURE

You are part of a grand design that is far beyond the grasp of modern science. In the simplest of terms, you are energy or spirit that's housed in your body. This divine energy that is God to most of us uses simple elements from the earth to form the complex organizations of plants, animals and humans. The process mostly remains a mystery and, outside of religious beliefs, most people don't give it much thought.

Try to imagine for a moment that your entire body was formed from a single microscopic cell. From that one single formless cell came trillions of living cells that make up the complex structures of your brain, eyes, muscles, bones every part of you. Somehow, all those cells still communicate and depend on each other. If you went another step further, you would find that inside each cell there are more living organisms at work with an intelligence that would stretch the limits of your imagination.

I don't mean to get philosophical; I just want you to grasp the magnitude of what you're dealing with. We are more complex than any computer or machine man will ever devise, just try to find a computer that can build, repair, or improve itself. The greatest minds throughout history have not even come close to understanding this awesome process.

Man will struggle to understand the mysteries of creation long after you're gone, but, for now, some facts are perfectly clear: your entire body is made from food, water, air, and light. This important fact is the basis of understanding human health, *for we truly are what we eat.*

Our bodies require over 60 known nutrients, some in amounts so small that we require only a few micrograms (millionths of a gram) each day, an amount too small to be seen without a microscope. Yet somehow this infinitesimal amount is distributed throughout your body and combined with other nutrients to create vital chemical reactions. This poorly understood orchestra of nutrition needs all of its players to work properly. If even a single one is missing, it will affect the function of all the others and you begin the slow suicide of degeneration.

Every year over 98% of your body is completely replaced entirely from the food you eat, the water you drink, and the air you breathe. The quality of your new cell structure will be determined by the quality of those nutrients. In two years, every cell in your body will have been replaced. That frightening thought should make it easier to reject the empty, processed, chemical concoctions that we dare to call food. With this in mind, let's see how our modern food supply stacks up.

"Eat to live, and not live to eat."

Benjamin Franklin

CHAPTER 3 - FOOD – WHAT'S IN IT FOR YOU?

In ancient times people had no choice but to eat the plants and animals that were native to the region in which they lived. The wisdom of nature is clear if you study the survival adaptations of plants and animals living in a particular area. Using the available nutrients, plants evolved for their best chance of survival in whatever climate they were growing in. The animals that ate those plants had those specialized nutrients available to them and they, in turn, also survived better. If that animal was then eaten, its flesh would also contain those nutrients. That's the food chain in a nutshell.

Prior to modern times, the vitamins, minerals, proteins, and fats that we needed to be healthy had been hidden in our food. Driven by our appetites, we never had to worry about the rest.

Our food is different now. Before the age of modern agriculture, farmers returned essential nutrients back to the soil. Manure for fertilizer, crop rotation, mulching and resting the land are practices that date back to ancient times.

After World War II, drug companies were faced with huge stockpiles of chemicals that were originally destined for the manufacture of bombs. They were able to convince American farmers that those chemicals could be used as a cheap fertilizer and ushered in the age of industrial farming. This was only about 55 years ago.

Today's crops are grown with just three minerals (**N**) Nitrogen, (**P**) Phosphorus, and (**K**) potassium). **NPK** fertilizers and over farming have damaged our farmlands. Most of the 60 or more essential minerals required for human health have been depleted from the soil. The crops may look just fine, but they are mineral deficient. Since your body cannot make minerals, you eventually become mineral deficient too.

In an effort to further increase crop yields, scientists have genetically engineered plants to grow better with the NPK fertilizer. These new crop strains have proven to be nutritionally inferior to wild strains because plants rely on minerals from the soil to make the chemical compounds they need. Many of those compounds are the nutrients we're hoping to get by eating them. Today's crops, grown on mineral deficient soils, don't contain all the nutrients they did just two generations ago.

Sadly much of the remaining nutrients are lost to the practices of modern food processing and storage. Here are just a few examples:

- 60-90% of vitamin B6 is lost in cereal milling and meat processing.
- Vitamin C is destroyed by heat and oxygen.
- Vitamin E is lost during storage and processing.

- 50% of folic acid can be lost during food preparation, processing and storage
- 80% of magnesium is lost in making white and enriched flours.
- Grapes lose up to 30% of their B vitamins, and asparagus loses 90% of its vitamin C after just one week in cold storage.
- Freezing meat can destroy 50% of vitamin B1 and B2, and 70% of vitamin B5.
- Cooking takes a further toll on nutrient losses.

Considering that the above list represents fresh fruits and vegetables, imagine the condition of the processed chemically altered junk foods that is consumed by most Americans. Virtually devoid of nutrients, processed foods provide empty calories that will fatten you up like a thanksgiving turkey.

Speaking of turkey, the meat you eat hasn't escaped the bastardization of mass production. The commercialization of feed animals has created fat and sick livestock that will, of course, ultimately make you fat and sick if you don't watch what you're doing. For example, most wild game carries only about 3-5% body fat on a natural diet. This includes deer, moose, sheep, pigs and cattle. Their domesticated counterparts carry 20-40% body fat. Pork can go as high as 60% fat. The fattest pigs are so unhealthy that it's not uncommon to lose a few animals to heart attacks during transport. Most feed animals are bred and fed deliberately to be fat because they are sold by the pound. You don't want to suffer the same fate. Natural free-range meats are available, so start to look for them.

If you are thinking that all this hasn't affected you, guess again. Large government sponsored surveys have shown that over 60% of the population is deficient in one or more of the essential nutrients. These surveys only measured for the minimum daily requirements (RDAs), not the optimum levels required for good health, nor was there any accounting for the increased requirements of athletics, stress, disease, pregnancy, lactation, or individual biological differences. Only 13 of the most common nutrients were tested for. If the remaining 47 or more essential nutrients are included, some form of deficiency is certain for almost everyone, and that probably includes you. Other surveys have shown deficiency ranges as high as 95% for certain nutrients.

A prolonged deficiency of any nutrient leads to progressive degeneration that can ultimately end in death if adequate amounts are not returned to the diet. The major degenerative diseases of today and Americas current battle of the bulge can be directly linked to poor nutrition.

The good news is that you can easily overcome the shortcomings of our modern day food supply. With the right nutritional supplementation, the knowledge to avoid empty foods, and just a little *wiggle*, you can go from fat and tired to lean and mean for the rest of your life.

The general public is just waking up to the fact that our mega food industry has ignored our health for the sake of profit. Degenerative diseases that once only affected the elderly now plague the middle aged. We will see the effects of our degraded food supply at younger and younger ages with each new generation.

"Because we don't think about future generations, they will never forget us."

Henrik Tikkanen

CHAPTER 4 - POISONS

It's clear that we are not receiving optimum amounts of essential nutrients from our food. This comes at a time when our bodies need extra nutrition in order to deal with a multitude of poisons that wouldn't normally be found in our food or environment.

Pharmaceutical drugs, chlorinization of water, industrial pollution of our soil, water and air, synthetic chemicals in paints, cleaners, glues, to name a few, have presented our systems with chemicals that can have disastrous effects on our health. The invisibility of these pollutants has lead to their acceptance in our everyday lives.

Highly toxic herbicides are sprayed along the roadsides all over this country just to keep the weeds down. They are likely carcinogens, can cause birth defects, are dangerous eye and skin irritants, and are highly mobile. That's an extreme price to pay, not to have to mow some grass. I'll bet you weren't aware you were being exposed to such dangerous practices.

Our food also carries a toxic burden. Because crops grown on depleted soils don't have the nutrients available to make the chemical compounds that discourage insects from eating them, farmers are forced to rely more and more on pesticides to protect their crops. Many of these pesticides, have shown conclusively to cause cancer, yet, they are still in use. Even when they are banned, many of these harmful chemicals are marketed to other countries. We then import the crops and end up ingesting the pesticides anyway.

The underlying theme of this book is that "you are what you eat." What you eat is built into your flesh, and, unfortunately, this includes toxins.

- A study commissioned by the World Wildlife Fund discovered that every person tested in the United Kingdom had detectable levels of potentially harmful man-made chemicals in their blood.

- Approximately 2.6 billion pounds of pesticides are sprayed on America each year. That's tens pounds for every single human being in the U.S.!

- There are over 50,000 pesticide products in use. Many have shown conclusively to cause cancer in experimental studies. The residues of these chemicals are found in produce.

- 90% of America's farmland is contaminated with pesticides.

- The U.S. Department of Public Health has warned that 85% of American drinking water is contaminated.

- In 1994 the FDA announced that the number of deaths in America from the "normal" use of prescription drugs is estimated at 150,000 people a year.

- More than half of the 15 million pounds of antibiotics made each year in the U.S. is used on livestock and poultry.

- 95% of poultry, 90% of pigs and 60% of cattle have antibiotics routinely added to their feed. The residues of these drugs are in the meat you eat.

- The overuse of antibiotics have bred drug-resistant bacteria which are also present in meat.

- It normally takes 16 weeks to raise a chicken. Using drugs, today's farmers can do it in just 6 weeks. Residues of those hormones are in the meat.

- 90% of swordfish are contaminated with mercury. 50% of white fish and 40% of salmon are contaminated with PCBs. Tragically, you may not have to concern yourself with this much longer. A new much publicized study in the journal *Nature* has estimated that industrial fishing has eliminated 90% of the populations of the world's big fishes.

You should also be aware of what is being fed to livestock since it will eventually end up in you. Animals also are what they eat, and toxins, as well as nutrients, follow the food chain.

Rendering plants are facilities that produce animal feed from the dead bodies and body parts of other animals. Because livestock are vegetarian animals, they are not equipped to deal with animal proteins. This feeding practice can lead to the production of an abnormal protein found in species involved in cannibalism and is the cause of "Mad Cow Disease." The protein can be transmitted to humans and is not destroyed by cooking. In England 2.5 million cows had to be destroyed to protect the public, yet the same feeding practices go on here. "Mad Cow Disease" has now been found in the U.S. and Canada. The disease has probably been here for some time. The illness does not usually show up in young animals and the disease can remain dormant for years, while most cattle are slaughtered before the age of four. Again, you're mostly on your own in protecting yourself, beef industry exports exceed 500 billion dollars a year, and they're not going down without a fight.

Salmon farms, which now supply most of the fresh salmon sold worldwide, have just recently come under attack. Farmed salmon, which supplies over 80% of America's third favorite seafood is so toxic with cancer causing chemicals that the Environmental Protection Agency recommends that you eat it less than once a month, and that pregnant women not eat it at all. Researchers confirmed that the problem is in the feed fed to the penned fish. Thanks to over fishing, wild salmon is extremely rare and there are no laws that require labeling whether the salmon are wild or farm raised.

According to *U.S. News and World Report,* cattle farmers are increasingly using chicken manure in feed. Researchers are experimenting with food garbage, fat from restaurant fryers, cattle and hog manure and even human sewage sludge for animal feed. (Yum!)

There's been recent talk about expanding the use of food irradiation to combat bacterial contamination. This may sound like a good idea until you take a closer look. The irradiation of food produces loads of toxic compounds not found in nature.

Consider that 500-1000 Rads of radiation will kill an adult human from the cellular damage it produces, and 100,000-20,000,000 Rads are used to irradiate food. You can be sure that your body is going to have no idea what to do with that chemical mess. Trust me, if bacteria can't live on it, neither can you. If you have children keep a close watch on this issue, it is currently being pushed in our school lunch programs.

There are hundreds of processed products on the market that contain artificial colorings, flavorings, preservatives and other additives not found in nature. They interfere with the delicate natural workings of our bodies, because they don't fit the highly specific requirements of our systems. Hidden fats, sugars, salt, and chemicals will take their toll on your health, so do your best to avoid them.

Probably the saddest example of all, are the Inuit people living in the artic. Long believed to be the healthiest people on the planet because of their rich diet of fresh seafood, and pristine environment, they live today much as their ancestors have for hundreds of years. Heart disease, cancer, diabetes and degenerative diseases had been virtually unknown to this people. Yet, our excesses have managed to invade even this innocent part of the world. Unknown to these hearty people, northbound winds have carried toxic remnants of faraway lands to their hunting grounds. As a result, their bodies contain the highest human concentrations of industrial chemicals and pesticides found anywhere on earth – levels so extreme that the breast milk and tissues of some Greenlanders could be classified as hazardous waste.

So it's official. We have polluted the entire planet, and about the only thing you can do about it is build up the resistance of your own body. That means supplementing your diet with the right nutrition and avoiding more pollutants. Read the program portion of this book carefully, and make sure you understand it. I have provided you with an easy way to start protecting yourself.

"If you violate Nature's laws you are your own prosecuting attorney, judge, jury, and hangman."

Luther Burbank

CHAPTER 5 - WE'RE GETTING FATTER

It might be easy to ignore the problems we've just looked at because they're not visible to the naked eye. It's harder to ignore what's visible to the eye of the naked, bodyfat. Have you ever stopped to wonder how it's possible that over half of the adults in the U.S. are overweight, when practically everyone would rather be thin? Surprisingly, the biggest increases are in young men and women ages 25-30. They're a full 10 lbs heavier today than they were just 15 years ago: Not taller, just fatter. All brought about from eating calories that are devoid of nutrients.

WHY ARE WE GETTING SO FAT?

It is the lack of nutrients, *not* excess calories that's fueling America's fat epidemic. Even though our portions are getting larger, it's estimated that obesity is the result of gross overeating in only about 10% of the cases, so excess calories alone cannot be the culprit. Under normal conditions, your body has mechanisms to deal with excess calories by raising your metabolic rate, burning more fat and glucose for fuel, inhibiting fat storage and, most importantly, quenching your appetite.

The nutrient content of your food is closely monitored by your brain, and for good reason. If a particular nutrient is deficient or missing, the biological processes that require it cannot take place. Every movement, thought, or cellular action you have depends on nutrients to take place. This is far more important from moment to moment than the energy required from calories. Even very lean people have enough stored energy in fat and muscle to run several marathons.

Scurvy is an example in which a simple vitamin C deficiency can lead to a painful death. Unable to produce the collagen that holds our tissues together, your body literally falls apart. A prolonged vitamin B12 deficiency causes nerve damage, insanity and eventually death. A selenium deficiency results in heart disease. It would fill an entire book to examine all the known diseases directly caused by nutritional deficiencies. A summary of vitamin and mineral functions and deficiencies can be found in the appendix at the back of this book.

Your appetite is driven by your body's need for nutrients. Due to the state of our modern food supply, your brain believes you are starving, while at the same time you're getting excess calories. This puts your body in an ideal state to put on fat. Your appetite goes up, your metabolism slows down, and you store fat more efficiently. By effectively reversing your normal responses, you have no chance of burning off the extra calories.

Empty calories will not only make you fat, they will also shorten the time you get to spend on this planet. In reputable scientific experiments, rats that were placed on calorie-restricted diets with adequate nutrient intake increased their life spans by 50%. It wasn't the reduced calorie level that gave the rats their extended life spans, it was the increased nutrient concentration per calorie. Today, we are experiencing just the opposite.

Think about this the next time you eat. So many commonly consumed foods contain almost zero nutrition, just a bunch of calories. The empty foods that make up the diets of the gravitationally-challenged, are also robbing their bodies of existing nutrients just to process them. Once you deplete your nutrient reserves, you are set up for all kinds of trouble. We often joke about a belly "that's all paid for," or "a little junk in the trunk," but it is no laughing matter. The commercial exploitation of our natural attraction for sweet, salty and fat is super sizing America. Empty calories from nutrient poor foods are responsible for our current fat epidemic, and it's making us sick to boot.

WHAT ARE WE DOING ABOUT IT?

The problem has been approached with the same mixed up medical mentality that keeps treating symptoms instead of the causes. Currently, Americans spend $35 billion annually on weight loss products and are getting fatter, not thinner. In spite of fad diets, fat burning formulas, celebrity endorsements and money back guarantees, the percentage of overweight adults has doubled since 1991.

Recently, the government commissioned the FDA to investigate the claims of all the popular weight loss programs. Their conclusion was that there was no evidence that any of them had much of a chance for long-term success. The public is presented with reports of a few individual successes, while most people gain back any lost weight. Now they are required to tell you so in their ads. What they don't have to tell you is that these programs may be setting you up to get even fatter, permanently!

We're all familiar with the famous definition of insanity. Doing something that doesn't work over and over again, and expecting a different result. If you're looking for a quick fix, you're not going to find one, so stop wasting your time, money, and health looking for a short cut.

If you're not getting the nutrients you need, you will never be able to stop overeating. The upside is that you can stop blaming your lack of willpower. With the right supplementation and better food choices, this is a very treatable condition.

ARE WE REALLY EATING THAT MUCH?

You bet! Most Americans have no idea how many useless calories that they put in their bodies each day. Using the government's recommendation of 2000 calories to meet your daily energy requirements, let's see how fast food adds up. An order of Burger Kings fries has 600 calories and a whopping 30 grams of fat. They may look like a side order, but from a calorie standpoint they're like burgers in disguise. A Quarter Pounder with cheese gives you the same 600 calories and almost all the fat. The Double Whopper with Cheese is the "king" (pun intended) at 1150 calories. When you add the soft drink, the value meals at fast food restaurants range between 1000 and 1800 calories. A bucket of movie theater popcorn is around 1600 calories, and a large order of cheese fries can be as high as 3000 calories. That's a lot of extra calories when you consider that you should be shooting for about 500 per meal. With all of those calories containing almost no nutrition, you can bet you'll be wearing them.

It's mind boggling to think that you could consume almost a full day's amount of calories in one meal and not get any nutrition. Instead, you've just loaded your body with heart-stopping saturated fat and empty calories.

DIETING WILL MAKE YOU FATTER

Almost all popular diets rely on reducing your food intake to 800-1200 calories per day. This is well below your body's daily energy requirement, so you use stored body fat and muscle for fuel. The result is usually rapid weight loss and the program would appear to be a success.

This predictable outcome has been exploited by the diet industry for decades. You pay your money, lose some weight, and tell a friend. What they don't tell is that you'll gain the weight back - and you will! Instead you're led to believe that you had lacked the will power to stay with the program, and you start again. These types of programs can't work no matter how they are disguised. Here's a look at the main reasons why, so you won't fall for them.

First, most low-calorie diets don't provide enough of the essential nutrients. We already know that this will slow your metabolism until, eventually, it will be very difficult to lose any more weight. A lack of essential nutrients will also fuel the cravings that will cause you to fail.

Second, muscle can provide up to 50 percent of the energy deficit on a low calorie diet. This is of major importance because muscle is where you burn most of your fat. Every ounce of muscle you lose reduces your ability to burn fat and lowers your metabolic rate. When you regain the weight, you don't regain the lost muscle, and that puts you on the fast track to getting even fatter.

Third, nature has equipped us with defenses against rapid weight loss by increasing your appetite, slowing your metabolism, and storing fat more effectively. If you've been at a particular weight for some time, that level of bodyfat becomes your *fat point*. If you lose weight too quickly, you will activate your body's defenses.

The most potent of these is an evolutionary enzyme called **lipoprotein lipase**. This enzyme is activated whenever we experience rapid fat loss. Its sole purpose is to quickly replenish your fat reserves. Obviously, this would be important in times of an uncertain food supply, but it is the archenemy of the modern dieter. Once activated, this enzymes job is to collect fat from your bloodstream and stuff it into your fat cells. It's so effective that it even reduces your ability to burn fat for energy, forcing your body to burn even more muscle while you are on your diet.

In the end, these mechanisms become so effective that when you finally crack and eat again, you can gain back all the weight that took you weeks of suffering to lose, in just a few days.

It is medically impossible for quick weight loss schemes to have lasting results, and repeated dieting can have long-term consequences. After enough failed attempts, you will eventually have lost so much muscle, and become so efficient at storing fat, that you may never be able to eat normally again.

If the idea of paying for two seats on your next plane ride doesn't sound appealing, read on and I'll show you how to work with your body to take off the weight and keep it off.

SO YOU'RE A LITTLE OVERWEIGHT?

You can rest in the knowledge that it has not been entirely your fault. Nutrient- poor food, inaccurate information, and the lure of a quick fix are all to blame. However, with that said, you need to be aware of the potential risks of sticking your head in the sand.

Americans are not just getting fatter, they are ballooning into extreme obesity. Obesity is generally defined as being about 30 pounds overweight. The number of extremely obese adults – those who are at least 100 pounds overweight has quadrupled since the 1980s to about 4 million. What was once thought to be a rare condition due to hormonal abnormalities has proven to be a combination of lifestyle factors and genetics. So while a few unfortunate souls are born with a body that is hyper-efficient at storing calories, many more are needlessly being created through poor nutrition and repeated dieting.

Excess body fat impairs your immune system, leaving you more susceptible to everything, and greatly increases your risk for cardiovascular disease, cancer, and diabetes. Interestingly, these are the same three killers most closely associated with nutritional deficiencies. You shouldn't be surprised!

If you are just moderately overweight your chance of developing diabetes doubles. If you are carrying an extra 60 pounds, you are 30 times more at risk.

Over a million people a year in this country have heart attacks. Often, there are no prior symptoms.

Childhood obesity has become a disturbing trend and the early signs of heart disease have been found in almost all children over the age of ten. I hope this is sinking in; we're not even giving our children a fighting chance.

The price of all this excess bodyfat is enormous, and is largely responsible for our current healthcare crisis. There have even been rumors of lawsuits against fast food purveyors similar to those against tobacco.

"We shall find the truth when we examine the problem. The problem is never apart from the answer. The problem is the answer - understanding the problem dissolves the problem."

Bruce Lee

NUTRIENTS – WHAT YOU NEED TO KNOW

You have to know what complete nutrition is, if you are going to do anything about getting it. Avoid the latest and greatest scams, or the next-cure all miracle nutrients. Recognize that you need them all, because they all work together. Here is a simple outline of what we'll be covering to help you keep the big picture in mind while we cover some of the details.

There are five parts consisting of:

- **PROTEIN**
- **ESSENTIAL FATS**
- **VITAMINS**
- **MINERALS**
- **CARBOHYDRATES**

Proteins, essential fats, vitamins, and minerals are the raw materials your body uses to build things, while carbohydrates supply the energy.

CHAPTER 6 - PROTEIN

When you think of protein you probably think of muscles, but proteins do so much more. Besides water, protein is the most plentiful substance in your body and is the structural component of every one of your cells. Your muscles, brain, organs, enzymes, immune system, and even your genes are built from proteins.

Proteins are made up of building blocks called amino acids. There are 21 different amino acids. All but 9 of them your body can make. The rest must come from your food. Your body uses different combinations of amino acids make to the multitude of different proteins it needs. A complete protein is one that contains all 21 amino acids.

Research has shown that short amino acid sequences can carry messages in our bodies. Some of these are formed during digestion when whole proteins are broken down. This helps explain why mixes of individual amino acids didn't work as expected when scientists tried to formulate better proteins for athletes. Again, nature knows best.

The quality of a protein is determined by its amino acid content and Biological Value (BV). The BV measures the amount of protein your body retains, by how much protein you have absorbed from your diet. Whole egg sets the standard score of 100. Other BV scores are: 80 for beef, 79 for chicken, 77 for casein, a protein found in milk, and 74 for soy.

As you can see, most whole foods are pretty much the same, so BV scores are really only important when choosing a protein supplement. Most protein supplements are made by isolating proteins from milk, egg, or soy. Whey protein concentrates have BV scores well over the 100 mark, and can be as high as 160. Additionally, studies have shown that whey protein may enhance your immunity by as much as 500%, while other proteins don't show this effect. With so many protein supplements on the market it's important to know what you are spending your hard earned money on. Choose a high quality whey protein first, egg protein second and leave the rest.

HOW MUCH PROTEIN?

If you've been eating the typical American diet, it's likely that you're not getting enough protein and getting way too much carbohydrate and fat. It is important that you know approximately what your personal protein requirement is so you can plan your diet around it. Too little protein and your body will cannibalize your muscle tissue to meet your protein needs. The resultant loss of lean body mass will reduce your metabolic rate and your ability to burn fat. Surplus protein is broken down into carbohydrates and urea. So, excess protein can make you fat, and high levels of urea can inflame your kidneys and cause low back pain. Of course, these are the extremes and our systems are not this strict. However, you should have some idea of what you're shooting for.

Use the table below to determine your approximate daily protein need, based on your lean body weight. Then do your best to include that amount in your diet.

Lean body weight = Actual wt. - (% body fat x actual wt.)

For example, if you weigh 180 lbs and are 25% body fat, take your body weight 180 pounds, times your percent body fat .25 to determine how much your fat weighs. In this case, it is 45 pounds. Now, just take your body weight of 180 pounds and subtract your fat weight of 45 pounds to get your lean body weight of 135 lbs. Use your lean body weight on the chart below to determine your approximate protein requirement.

Just get close. Unless you're a professional athlete, you'll be just fine. The point here is that fat doesn't do anything, so you don't need to feed it.

The estimates given below are based on a moderate workout schedule.

LEAN BODYWEIGHT	DAILY PROTEIN REQUIREMENT (grams)
100	68
120	82
140	96
160	109
180	123
200	136
220	150
240	164

Getting enough protein is a bigger deal for athletes. Exercise greatly increases your protein needs, and, if you're not getting enough, you'll be missing a lot of the benefits of your hard work. If you've been training with heavy weights, take your protein requirements seriously.

WHAT YOU NEED TO REMEMBER

Animal products provide complete proteins, meaning that they supply all the amino acids your body requires. Pick lean sources like chicken, turkey, fish, shellfish, and egg whites. Try to limit your intake of meats high in saturated fats like beef and pork.

If you're a vegetarian it's more difficult to meet your protein needs because most plant sources don't contain the full complement of amino acids. Make sure you mix your protein foods throughout the day, and use a supplement.

When choosing a protein supplement, use a high quality whey protein concentrate. It has the highest biological value and can boost your immune system. Egg white protein is second best. Avoid cheaper proteins like casein and protein blends where you can't be sure of what you're getting. Use soy protein in moderation, since it has a low biological value, and may have some effects on thyroid and hormone metabolism.

Regardless of what your protein requirement turns out to be, you can only absorb about 30-35 grams per meal under normal conditions. If you have higher requirements you will have to plan more meals.

CHAPTER 7 - ESSENTIAL FATS

There are many different kinds of fats. Your body can make all but two of them from protein and carbohydrates. That's why even though fat is your main source of fuel, you don't need to eat very much of it. You need to eat fat to obtain the two fats our bodies can't make. They are the **Essential Fatty Acids (EFAs), Linoleic Acid** and **Alpha Linolenic Acid.** From these two fats, your body can make every other kind of fat it needs.

Essential fatty acids are not burned for fuel. They are built into your cells and are found in especially high concentrations in the specialized structures of your eyes, ears, brain, adrenal glands, and sex organs.

Here is a look at some of what medical science has uncovered about these special fats:

- EFAs provide the raw material for a family of powerful hormone-like substances that control the physiological actions of your body on a moment to moment basis.

- EFAs are involved in making oxygen available to body tissues. They also appear to hold oxygen in our cell membranes where it acts as a barrier to viruses, bacteria, and fungi that cannot thrive in its presence.

- EFAs substantially shorten the time required for fatigued muscles to recover from exercise.

- At levels above 15% of your total calories, they increase your metabolic rate and increase the use of stored bodyfat. Essential fats will help keep you thin.

- EFAs help carry toxins to the surface of the skin, intestines, kidneys, and lungs to be discarded out of the body.

- They may play a part in chromosome stability, and may have functions in starting and stopping gene expression.

- EFAs are required for normal brain development in children, and are essential for healthy skin.

- Alpha linolenic acid improves stamina, speeds healing, reduces inflammation, alleviates PMS, decreases arthritis pain, and inhibits tumor growth.

- EFAs play a role in preventing heart disease, cancer, and diabetes

There is no mistaking the importance of essential fats to our health. The problem is that, like most natural foods, essential fats don't have a very good shelf life. They are easily destroyed when exposed to light, heat, and oxygen. Modern food processing, storage, and cooking have made essential fats scarce in today's diet.

To make matters worse, many commonly consumed foods can interfere with essential fatty acid metabolism in the body. The worst offenders are partially hydrogenated oils, sugars, and saturated fats.

Processed and partially hydrogenated oils are particularly damaging because they contain unnatural fats that your body tries to make use of when EFAs are absent. They end up being built into your cells, resulting in abnormal cell function and leaky cell membranes that allow toxins to enter. These nasty fats have been implicated in both cardiovascular disease and cancer.

Sugar and refined carbohydrates raise your insulin levels, which inhibits the release of stored EFAs from your bodyfat. Sugar carries a lot more bad news for your body, but more on that later.

Changes in our fat consumption and the accompanying destruction of EFAs from processing, heating and hydrogenation are probably responsible for more human disease than anything else I will write about in this book.

WHAT YOU NEED TO REMEMBER

Essential fats are probably deficient in your diet. They will not make you fat but, instead, help to make you thin. Do your best to avoid most other fats, especially partially hydrogenated oils. Look for them on labels as they are in almost every processed food.

The best sources of EFAs are Flax seed oil, and other seed oils such as pumpkin seed, borage oil, and evening primrose oil. Be sure that they are organic, cold pressed, unprocessed oils or they lose their healthy properties. Supplementing with an organic flax seed oil blend is inexpensive insurance to make sure you are getting a good supply of these important fats. As always, the important functions of essential fats require other nutrients to perform properly.

Fish oils are a rich source of preformed EFAs. However, they cannot be trusted for freshness and have a high probability of containing toxins, and so should be reserved for those few individuals with enzyme deficiencies.

NOTE: Essential fatty acid requirements may be increased in times of decreased sunlight and cold weather. If you live in northern latitudes or the Pacific Northwest this information is even more important in wintertime.

CHAPTER 8 - PROTEIN AND OIL WORK TOGETHER

We have examined protein and essential fats (EFAs) separately, but you don't want to eat them that way. Protein and essential fats are found together in whole foods, natural meats, and in your body. They work together to provide the main structural components of all the cells in your body.

In experiments, researchers have observed that if just protein is given to animals deficient in essential fats, the animals die very quickly. In another experiment done over 100 years ago, starving dogs that were provided either only protein or only fat died faster than if they were given no food at all. In other words they continued to starve. When they were fed protein and fat together, they quickly recovered from starvation.

This information has to be interpreted a little differently today, but is still relevant. Protein sources of the past, like free-range livestock, wild game, and whole grains all contained EFAs. So, if you were getting adequate protein, you were probably also getting essential fats. Today's grains are stripped of their EFA content. Beef can be up to 40% saturated fat and contains almost no essential fats. Poultry is only a little better. Because there are no EFAs in their feed, there are no EFAs in their flesh. The same goes for you.

The nutritional industry sells protein supplements that contain almost no fat. They would be much more effective if essential fats were added. You are also less likely to suffer from protein related food allergies when EFAs are present. You won't find this combination in the same container regardless of what the label says. Oils containing EFAs have to be specially prepared and kept refrigerated.

Protein and essential fat combinations have been used as a natural remedy to effectively treat liver disease, and have shown promise in treating cancers and reducing tumor growth. More research needs to be done for sure, but for now we would be wise to follow nature's example.

WHAT YOU NEED TO REMEMBER

Proteins and essential fats are cellular building blocks in our bodies. Taken together, they will improve your health and aid in fat loss.

Diets high in saturated fats and low in EFAs can cause obesity and fatty degeneration. The same is true for a diet high in refined carbohydrates. Unfortunately, this is representative of how the typical American eats.

CHAPTER 9 - VITAMINS

Vitamins are not food. They are components of food that enable the proteins, fats, and carbohydrates to work in our bodies. They are the co-factors that facilitate many of the chemical reactions that take place in our bodies, and are also involved in the cleaning up of the by-products of those reactions. Vitamins are involved in the processes of building, repairing, and protecting every one of our cells.

Vitamins help regulate your metabolism, and make possible the conversion of carbohydrates and fats to energy. This provides yet another example of how our modern food supply can fatten you up. Most processed foods are, by and large, carbohydrate and fat. Because these empty foods don't contain the necessary vitamins for your body to process them, each time you eat these foods you rob your body of any existing vitamins and, make yourself even more deficient. You end up with high calories and a slow metabolism, and that doesn't paint a pretty picture for your waistline.

Stress, exercise, illness, pregnancy, alcohol, smoking, and exposure to toxins all increase your vitamin requirements. Nutritional supplements have shown great benefit in easing the withdrawal from drugs and alcohol, and are mandatory for getting over food addictions. Interestingly, it's usually the people who need the additional nutrition the most that are least likely to seek it out. Then, in a sad twist of fate, those nutrient deficiencies help perpetuate their bad habits and addictions. Forward thinking clinicians will find that enhanced nutrition will benefit many disorders.

I hope you're starting to see a pattern developing here. Without proper nutrition, your mind and body can't function properly. There is abundant evidence that the solutions to preventing many birth defects, degenerative diseases, and others curses you think may have been brought upon you by fate, is to ensure an optimal intake of nutrients.

Except for a limited few, our bodies cannot make vitamins, hence, we must get them in our food. Our modern food supply has let us down again, and it no longer contains sufficient amounts of vitamins to maintain optimum health.

Like all nutrients, vitamins interact with each other, and also require minerals to work properly. Haphazard vitamin supplementation is common, but won't do you much good. First, you must establish a complete baseline plan that includes all of the essential nutrients. Then, you can begin to fine-tune your intake of nutrients to suit your biochemical individuality or special needs. Vitamins don't stay in your system long and need to be continually replaced everyday. When you do it right, you'll feel the difference.

NOTE: For information on the functions of the individual vitamins and symptoms associated with their deficiencies, see appendix.

Until you return to the ground since from it you were taken;
for dust you are and to dust you shall return.

-GENESIS 3 19

CHAPTER 10 - MINERALS

There are 79 minerals that have been detected in human and animal tissue. At least 60 of these have proven to be essential to human health. Some are required in gram amounts and some in amounts so small that you could not see them on the head of a pin (millionths of a gram). Yet somehow your body separates out those few molecules and transports them to the cells where they become the very currency of health.

Minerals are involved in virtually everything you do. They are even necessary for you to utilize vitamins. If vitamins are absent, your body can still make some use of minerals. However, without minerals, vitamins are totally useless. Organically not a single function in your body can take place with out at least one mineral co-factor.

The interaction between minerals in our bodies is complex. Take your bones for example. To build bone, requires you have enough calcium, magnesium, silicon, fluoride, zinc, copper, boron, manganese, phosphorus, vitamin D, protein, hormones, and pressure. Without them all, nothing happens. It's obvious that even a mountain of just calcium won't do a thing to prevent osteoporosis, but it's still the most common advice given.

Concern over the mineral content of our farmlands is not a new subject. In 1936, U.S. Senate Document 264 reported on the depletion rates of the world's farm and range soils. In it, it was reported that the Earth's soils are anemic. In 1992, an Earth Summit Report was issued, adding support to what was reported so much earlier. The decline in percentages of mineral values over the last hundred years was overwhelming. North American farm and range soils have been depleted by 85 percent. You won't be hearing a lot about this because there's really nothing that can be done to reverse what greed and ignorance has brought upon us. Our crops no longer contain the minerals necessary for human health, and we are paying the price in degenerative disease. Science will try to put a band-aid on the problem with genetically engineered crops and more drugs for you and your children. You, of course, will be charged handsomely for all the help. Isn't it funny how you never get a refund when it doesn't work?

Like vitamins, your body can't make minerals. You must get them from your food. Numerous nutritional assays have shown that you're probably not getting sufficient amounts of many minerals. The predictable result is progressive degenerative disease. Correcting a deficiency will usually reverse the symptoms, provided the organ has not been damaged beyond its ability to recover. Nobody knows where that mysterious point of no return is, so never write yourself off.

TRACE MINERALS (RARE EARTHS)

Calcium, magnesium, phosphorus, potassium, chloride, and sodium are minerals that you've probably heard of. They are macro-minerals that you require in larger amounts so they are better studied more talked about and. That doesn't make them any more or less important than trace minerals that you only need tiny amounts of. If just one of the essential minerals is not adequately supplied, the others can't function properly. They all work together, so it's crucial that you get a balanced supply.

Trace minerals are normally found in topsoil and the biological functions of many of these trace minerals are just being discovered. Because they occur in such small quantities it's difficult for scientists to study them. It was not long ago that minerals like selenium, chromium, vanadium, arsenic, nickel, and others, were thought to be totally toxic. Now they're accepted as essential nutrients. It's known today that our thyroid glands cannot make hormones without iodine, a selenium deficiency results in heart disease, a lithium deficiency can affect your personality, and chromium and vanadium help control blood sugar and prevent diabetes. These and many others have proven to be vitally important to our health.

Cravings, binging, and salt hunger are behaviors that can be traced to mineral deficiencies. Your body temporarily translates sugar and salt consumption as fulfillment of your need for nutritional minerals. This relationship has been well exploited by the snack and fast food industry. Interestingly, neither a vitamin deficiency, protein deficiency, nor calorie deficiency initiates this behavior, nor will vitamin supplements, eating carbohydrate, protein, or fat quench it.

Bizarre cravings are common in mineral starved animals and humans. Eating dirt and chewing ice, the chewing of cloth, hair, paint, calk, animal feces and other non-foods are signs of mineral deficiency. Pregnant women are legendary for their unusual cravings. In most cases, mineral supplementation will stop the behavior.

Suffice it to say that you should be supplementing with the trace minerals that would normally be found in the soil and in your food. *Plant derived colloidal minerals* are natural and highly absorbable. Don't be fooled by colloids made from clay, seawater, the Great Salt Lake, or the like. These are inorganic forms and are not well absorbed by your body. It should be obvious that we can't drink seawater or eat soil to get our minerals, but these are sold nonetheless.

Eating a healthy diet of fresh fruits, vegetables and whole grains is still good advice, but you can no longer trust their mineral content. Be honest: you're probably not doing that anyway, so you should be especially conscious to supplement.

TOXIC METAL ELIMINATION BY MINERAL SUBSTITUTION

Too much of a single mineral is just as detrimental to your health as too little. For instance, a tiny amount of arsenic is necessary for certain enzymes in your body. Receive too much and it can easily kill you. For this reason, minerals interact in our bodies to form a natural balance and prevent poisoning. Calcium is the recognized antidote for lead poisoning, and selenium is the antidote for mercury poisoning, if you take too much iron, it interferes with zinc metabolism and so on.

With the continuing industrial pollution of our food, water, and air by heavy metal contaminants, proper mineral supplementation is even more critical. For example, cadmium is a common industrial pollutant. It's also found in cigarette smoke and is easily absorbed when inhaled. If you're a nonsmoker, don't feel left out. There is plenty left for you in second-hand smoke. Cadmium interferes with a number of other minerals including zinc (weakened immune function, and decreased sexual function), copper (loss of skin elasticity and aneurysms), calcium (osteoporosis, arthritis, and hypertension), and selenium (heart disease, and cancer). We are just beginning to scratch the surface on how pollution and the lack of minerals in our food supply are affecting our physical and mental health. Make sure you get a good balance of minerals, and never take them singularly.

NOTE: For information on the functions of the individual minerals and the symptoms associated with their deficiencies, see appendix.

CHAPTER 11 - CARBOHYDRATE

Carbohydrates are basically sugars. The different forms of carbohydrates are determined by how the different sugar molecules are linked together. It's been estimated that the average Americans diet consists of 89% carbohydrate and fat.

Nothing in your body is made from carbohydrates. They are only burned for energy. If your body were an engine, carbohydrates would be the gas in the tank. If you try to add more fuel to an already full tank, the excess just spills out. In your body, sugar (glucose) is the fuel stored in your muscles and liver for quick bursts of energy, and is the preferred fuel for your brain. When your tank is full, the extra sugar spills over and builds up in your blood stream. High blood sugar is toxic to your system, and your body quickly cleans up the mess by converting the excess into fat and storing it for later use.

Athletes are like high performance engines. They burn much more fuel because of their higher energy requirements. For them, getting enough carbohydrates can mean the difference between victory and defeat. This is not so for most Americans, who consume a diet rich in refined carbohydrates and get little or no exercise. If you want to stay healthy and get lean, you have to adjust the type and amount of carbohydrates you consume to suit your body type and lifestyle.

Natural carbohydrates are found in whole grains, fresh vegetables, and fresh fruits. They are combined with fiber, oils, vitamins, and minerals, and are absorbed slowly, trickling in the energy as you need it while supplying you with essential nutrients.

Processed carbohydrates are quite different. Refined sugars and starches found in all processed foods have had their fiber, oils, vitamins, and minerals removed. They are absorbed too rapidly and flood your system with sugar that your body quickly turns into fat. Foods like white flour, white rice, pasta, enriched flours in breads (both white and dark), corn starch, breakfast cereals, white potatoes and products made with these ingredients will make you fat.

A study currently being done by Harvard Medical School is challenging the governments recommended food pyramid, which says that our diets should be high in starches, grains, cereals, rice and pasta. These foods have been proven to increase your cravings for more food. America's obsession with snack foods, soft drinks, breads and cereals far exceeds anyone's energy requirement. Snacking on sweets, soft drinks, fruit juices, pastries or baked goods can keep you storing fat all day long.

Our cravings for sweet foods were an evolutionary way for us to get the vitamins and minerals contained in fruits and vegetables. This important adaptation has been turned against you by the food industry and, now, sugar is added to just about everything, even meat. No doubt the evidence is "hanging over your belt."

WHAT YOU NEED TO REMEMBER

Carbohydrates are not really the enemy, just the form that most people eat them in. Complex carbohydrates are essential for short-term energy and helps spare muscle protein. For athletes this can mean the difference between winning and losing. The less you exercise, the less carbohydrate you can tolerate. So, be realistic about your activity level. Get your carbohydrates from whole grains, fresh vegetables, and seasonal fruits, and eat them raw whenever possible.

If it comes in a bag or a box, or has been puffed or processed, it's a safe bet it's not good for you. Sugar and refined carbohydrates will not only make you fat, but are also linked to heart disease, cancer, diabetes and many other potential health problems. Because they have been stripped of their nutrients, processed foods rob your body of existing nutrients. Sugared drinks, including fruit juices, are the worst, they raise blood sugar levels highest of all. Eliminate them from your diet!

If you're overweight don't eat any refined carbs (bread, cereals, pasta, white rice, potatoes, etc.). You can and should still eat plenty of raw vegetables and some fruit. Keep in mind if you're eating salads, that most salad dressings are mainly processed fats that will ruin your healthy salad. Stick with vinegar and olive oil with spices.

NOTE: In an effort to avoid calories, many dieters have turned to artificial sweeteners.

Diet foods can be a major contributor to obesity. The reasons are not simple, they involve complex biochemical reactions linked to hormones and brain chemicals.

*For example the artificial sweetener **Aspartame**, also known as **NutraSweet** or **Equal** doesn't have any calories. However, one of its ingredients, the amino acid phenylalanine can interfere with the production of serotonin, a nerve chemical that among other things controls food cravings. A shortage of serotonin adversely affects your mood and will make your brain and body scream for the foods that create more of this brain chemical. Those foods are the high calorie, high carbohydrate foods that can sabotage your diet. Also the sweet taste prompts your body to produce insulin even though no food is entering your blood stream. The resultant drop in blood sugar fuels intense sugar cravings to restore blood sugar levels and a vicious cycle begins.*

Artificial sweeteners have been shown to have negative side affects on your blood sugar levels, your metabolism, and have even been shown to cause cancer. Avoid them, and leave your vices behind you.

Human happiness is produced not so much by pieces of good fortune that seldom happen, as by little advantages that occur everyday.

-Benjamin Franklin

CHAPTER 12 – LOSING IT THE RIGHT WAY

I could go on and on about health and nutrition, but experience tells me that the majority of you are looking for help losing weight. That's good because being overweight is one of your biggest health risks. The current healthcare cost of obesity is $117 billion per year, five times the costs associated with tobacco.

There are many factors involved in gaining and losing weight, including emotions, brain chemistry, hormones, stress, and self image, just to name a few. Don't let yourself get caught up in the complexity of this. Far and away, your biggest problems are your eating habits and our degraded food supply. Fortunately, almost everything else is in some way linked to your nutritional status anyway.

Even if you've failed before, you should have some idea where you may have gone wrong by the end of this book. You'll find that by following a few simple rules, you can take the weight off, keep it off, and improve your health to boot. This program is designed to replace bad habits one at a time until you're doing the right things unconsciously. At that point, it's not a program at all, and you'll have succeeded in making permanent lifestyle changes.

The very first thing you must do is change your views about losing weight. You have all the information you need to re-program yourself and avoid the quick weight loss scam.

Secondly, make your changes just a little at a time. Both your mind and body will rebel against drastic changes, even if they're good for you. Examples of this can be seen in the withdrawal symptoms experienced from alcohol, drugs, cigarettes and, yes, even food. Though some substances may be poisonous to your system, with long-term use your body makes adjustments to them that can make it very uncomfortable for you when they are removed from your daily routine. Whatever your present state, change one thing at a time and make it stick.

A good example is soft drinks. Sugared drinks are one of your greatest enemies, and the companies that make them have done everything they can to keep you addicted (just like the tobacco industry). If you do only one thing, eliminate soft drinks (this includes diet) and fruit juices. Drink pure water. It's not easy at first, but after a few weeks you won't miss it. You'll find that it's just as easy to make good choices as it is to make bad ones - they're just choices. Each change you make will build on the last one until, over time, it'll be mission accomplished and you'll have barely broken a sweat.

The following steps outline where you'll be headed. Don't try to incorporate all of them at once. It's tempting, but you'll be setting yourself up to fail. I'll show you how you can gradually incorporate these steps into permanent lifestyle changes.

This is the longest chapter of the book. Read it carefully because you need to know exactly what you're doing. Then you can forget the details and confidently get on board.

- **STEP 1:   Get your nutritional needs met.** If even one nutrient is missing or deficient, your body will continue to ask for it via your appetite, and your metabolism will slow down. Eventually, your health will suffer.

- **STEP 2:   Lose weight very slowly.** Lose no more than a half-pound per week, or you will excite your body's defense mechanisms and gain the weight back.

- **STEP 3:   Cut out the simple sugars.** Sweet drinks are the worst for spiking your blood sugar. Fruit juices are no substitute, ounce for ounce, orange juice contains more sugar than Coca-Cola. Processed carbohydrates such as those found in (rice cakes, most breads, pastries, crackers, and chips) also apply here. Watch for ingredients containing sugar, honey, or corn syrup.

- **STEP 4:   Cut back on all fats except essential fats.** Dry foods like crackers, chips and baked goods are loaded with fat. So are frozen desserts and salad dressings. Don't be fooled by low fat labels. Avoid margarines and shortenings found in almost all baked goods, and pass on the deep fried foods. Use a supplement to increase your intake of Essential Fatty Acids.

NOTE: In many instances step 3 and 4 are the same foods

- **STEP 5:   Don't skip meals.** Skipping meals makes you fatter by causing an insulin burst as soon as you eat again. The excess insulin is converted to fat and can more than make up for the skipped meal.

- **STEP 6:   Exercise 6 days per week.** You will lose three times as much fat compared to exercising 2-3 times per week regardless of the duration. More importantly, you'll be more likely to do it. Trying to start with 2 or 3 days a week is the ticket to quitting because you'll never establish a habit. Fit people think about activity everyday because it's fun. You will too.

Basically, if you supplement correctly, gradually make better food choices, and get some kind of physical activity, your body will do the rest.

That's it! Everyone can implement these simple habits to some degree, from the unhealthiest couch potato to the most elite athlete. The training may change, the nutritional requirements may be different, the goals may be loftier, but the principles are the same. Get your nutritional needs met, keep out the junk, and exercise. Then, watch your body change to your will.

The rest of this chapter is dedicated to expanding your knowledge of these principles, then all you have to do is get started!

STEP 1. - NUTRITION

Throughout this book, we have seen that almost all of our modern health problems and America's current fat epidemic are directly related to our degraded food supply. This isn't going to change any time soon, so to have any long-term success, you are going to need proper nutritional supplementation. Though we are all biochemically unique, everyone must first establish a nutritional base of protein, essential fats, vitamins, and minerals before you can even begin to explore what your unique nutritional needs might be.

Getting all your nutrients in adequate amounts and in the correct ratios to each other is a complex undertaking and requires knowledge that is beyond the scope of this book. The market place is full of supplements; some are good and some are completely useless. You have to be an expert to know the difference, and the same corporate greed that got us here in the first place is alive and well in the nutritional industry. The average American can't possibly find time to research vitamin and mineral formulas, and that leaves most people susceptible to every scam under the sun. The old adage" if it sounds too good to be true, it probably is" just doesn't seem to apply when you're desperate. That is why I started this project in the first place.

It took me years to come to the conclusions presented in this book. It was written to take the guesswork out of health and weight loss. For this same reason, I've developed a product to take the guesswork out of nutritional supplementation.

NUTRALL (all nutrients) is a meal replacement that's based on everything you've read so far. It will provide a quick and effective way to start your rebuilding program without worrying if all your bases are covered. Remember that every nutrient relies on others to function properly, and you need them every day. Without a sound nutritional base, you're destined for failure. It's where you must begin. You can read about **NUTRALL** in the appendix at the back of this book, or visit WWW.NUTRALL.COM or use the information to form your own supplement.

STEP 2 - GO SLOW

You've seen that quick weight loss practically guarantees that you'll regain the weight. We have an entire industry with a failure rate of over 95% to prove it. In order to lose bodyfat and still keep your muscle, you must take the weight off slowly, so that you won't alert your body's defense mechanisms. This means that you can't change your present calorie intake by very much. Start by focusing on improving your food choices while continuing to eat at your normal level. Some of you will have to eat more if you have been on a low calorie diet.

The most weight you can lose without alarming your body's defense mechanisms is only about a half pound of fat per week. With this in mind, plan accordingly. Trying to speed up the process won't work; you'll just gain it back.

Be aware that weight loss and fat loss may not be the same. You've seen that if you lose weight incorrectly, up to 50% of the lost weight can be from muscle. Since you're only interested in losing fat, and your body weight can fluctuate by pounds from day to day, scales are not a very good way to determine your progress. If you're concerned with your progress, have your body fat tested every few months to make sure you are losing fat. Methods of bodyfat testing vary, so use the same system every time.

When you begin to exercise with weights, you may initially put on muscle faster than you lose the fat. You'll look and feel leaner and your clothes will fit better, but you may not have lost any weight. For some women, the thought of increasing muscle size is a concern. Don't worry, women have only 1/10 the testosterone that men do so gaining muscle is more difficult for them. Fight to get any muscle you can, it will only accent your natural feminine curves and rev up your metabolism. Most of the masculine women you see in the magazines got that way through drug use. Real muscle looks good on everyone.

Finally, if your fat loss plateaus after establishing your nutritional base and changing some of your food choices, you can slowly begin to reduce your calorie intake. Don't cut out more than 300-400 calories per day, and keep it there until your fat loss plateaus again, don't rush it. Two pounds per month may seem like nothing at first, especially if you have a lot of weight to lose, but patience will pay off. In one year you'll have lost 25 pounds of fat that will stay off.

Your other alternative is to follow everyone else on idiotic diets and lose 25 pounds after a few months of starving yourself, half of which will be muscle. You'll have to eat again eventually, and, when you do, you'll quickly gain back all the fat you suffered to lose, plus a little extra. You won't gain back the muscle, and you'll be fatter and more unhealthy than you were before you started. I have just described the American diet industry and the uninformed can get roped in and ruin their metabolisms. Don't you be one of them.

Time waits for no one and the months will surely go by for all of us. Your only real decision is where you want to be one or two years from now. Don't get anxious for a quick fix, or you'll continually be starting over years from now.

DEADLY FOODS TO AVOID

STEP 3 - KILLER FATS

It's worth repeating that essential fats are required in your diet so *don't* avoid them. Instead, increase your intake of these special oils. They are healthy fats, and increasing them in your diet will help you lose body fat and improve your health.

With that said, you should try to avoid as much of other fats as possible. Your body can make all the fat it needs from essential fats and the conversion of protein and carbohydrates. Research shows conclusively that eating fat puts on bodyfat easier than other foods.

Body fat is not the only reason you should avoid most commercial fats and oils. Changes that occur during the processing and cooking of the fats that we commonly consume can lead to health problems far more frightening than unsightly bodyfat.

During the refining process natural healthy vegetable and seed oils have all of their protein, vitamin, and mineral content removed to extend their shelf-life. The end result is a product that is completely devoid of nutrients. This should sound familiar, since the food industry has done the same thing with grains to make flour. Creating yet another nutritionally empty food would be bad enough, but it gets worse. Many of these oils are then hydrogenated to make margarine and shortenings.

The hydrogenation process requires heating oils to high temperatures that unnaturally twist some of the essential fat molecules *(trans fatty acids)*, thus destroying their healthy properties. The process also creates large amounts of cell-damaging free radicals and many other toxic by-products.

Frying and deep-frying exposes oils to their three most damaging effects simultaneously (heat, light, and oxygen). Heat twists the molecules, light creates free radical reactions, and oxidation causes oils to go rancid (rotten).

Heated oils interfere with the vital functions of essential fats and worsen essential fatty acid deficiencies. The following are some of the adverse affects resulting from the over consumption of altered fats.

- Increased cholesterol levels
- Increased triglycerides levels (blood fat)
- Lowered immune response
- Decreased insulin sensitivity (insulin resistance)
- Altered cell membranes (leaky cells)
- Changes in size, number, and composition of fat cells.
- Affects future use of body fat
- Affects liver enzyme functions
- Decreases testosterone levels

It's no surprise that getting adequate amounts of essential fats does just the opposite.

The increase in consumption of hydrogenated and altered vegetable oils is closely correlated with the increase in cancer and heart disease that has occurred in the last century. Since these fats have detrimental effects on our cardiovascular system, immune system, reproductive system, liver function, essential fat metabolism, and energy production, I think that I can safely say that margarines, shortenings, partially hydrogenated oils, and deep frying are hazardous to your health and should be avoided.

The up side is that our bodies preferentially burn harmful fats for energy, and conserves essential fats for vital functions. Supplementation goes a long way if you can't always eat right.

STEP 4 - SUGAR

Sugar consumption in the United States has increased from 15 lbs per person a year in 1815 to over 155 lbs per person today. This huge increase in sugar consumption is wreaking havoc on our bodies.

When you consume sugar in excess of your body's energy requirements it's quickly turned into saturated fat (triglycerides) and carried by your blood to be stuffed away in your fat cells and organs. These blood fats interfere with the function of the hormone insulin, so you have to produce higher and higher amounts to control your blood sugar. High insulin levels don't allow you to use stored bodyfat for fuel and encourages your body to form new fat. If this condition persists over a long period of time your pancreas can become weakened from overuse. When your body can no longer produce enough insulin to control your blood sugar, you become diabetic. Complications resulting from type II diabetes is the third leading cause of death in the U.S.

Saturated fats also cause red blood cells to stick together. This decreases the supply of oxygen to body tissues, lowering your metabolism and making you feel lethargic.

Sugar inhibits your immune system, causes inflammation, and supports the development of food allergies. The symptoms of which can include, asthma, joint pain, muscle pain, colitis and some behavioral disorders. Food allergies have been implicated in the development of autoimmune diseases as well. I will explain this theory in more detail later.

Sugars put your body in a state of stress by increasing the production of adrenaline and cortisone. If this continues unabated, your adrenal glands become fatigued, and you can no longer respond to stress normally. Chronic fatigue, over eating, and weight gain are signs of adrenal weakness. High levels of cortisone suppress your immune system and cause stomach ulcers.

Sugar interferes with the function of vitamin C which can lead to accelerated aging and wrinkled skin.

Finally, processed sugars and starches lack the vitamins and minerals for their own metabolism, and eating them drains your body of its nutrient reserves. Sugar loads increase the normal rate of mineral loss in sweat and urine by 300 percent for up to 12 hours. There is no amount of supplementation that can keep up with this loss. Eating empty foods literally suck the nutrients right out of you. How much reserves you have are partially determined by your genetics, and the nutrients you get from your diet. It's Russian Roulette to push your luck.

STEP 5 - EAT ON SCHEDULE

In order to lose bodyfat and maintain your muscle, you must control your insulin levels. We recognize insulin as the hormone involved in controlling blood sugar levels; however, insulin is also necessary for muscle growth and, unfortunately, fat deposition. If you're confused on how you're going to gain muscle and lose fat, you're not alone. However, it's not as complicated as it seems.

The presence of insulin signals your body to store food energy preferably in your muscles and liver where it'll be available for immediate use. Once those are full, the rest goes to bodyfat. When you exercise, insulin combines with growth hormone and other nutrients to build lean muscle tissue, decreases body fat, and help replenish your energy stores.

The common practice of snacking on processed foods and sugared drinks while sitting around on your keester causes a rapid rise in blood sugar which spikes your insulin levels. If you haven't just finished a workout, all that sugar is promptly converted to fat and stored unflatteringly on your figure.

Excess insulin itself is toxic and is also converted to fat by your liver. The familiar practice of skipping meals in an effort to lose weight can actually make you fatter by causing insulin bursts when you eat again. The conversion of insulin to fat can more than make up for the missed calories from the skipped meal and is often exaggerated by the tendency to over eat at the next meal.

The key is to keep your insulin levels steady and get regular exercise. The easiest way is to eat 5 small meals per day instead of two or three big ones and pick whole foods that won't spike your blood sugar. This is pretty easy stuff once you get started. For example, drink water instead of sodas and fruit juice, eat an apple instead of a donut. You get the idea. Even if you frequent fast food restaurants, you could have the burger, but skip the fries and soft drink. In the beginning it takes a bit of will power to get past the meal deal brain washing, but after a while it will be second nature, and you'll have saved a load of cash.

STEP 6 - EXERCISE

I must begin this section with a little tough love. If you're not interested in doing a little regular exercise, start praying, because you're going to need a miracle. The human body is a machine that breaks down when you don't use it. The mechanisms maintaining our bodies rely on activity. Bones need pressure to stay strong. Stress on our muscles makes them stronger. Muscle contractions help push blood back to our hearts. Movement lubricates our joints. Learning and problem solving keep our brains sharp. Even your hormones require regular exercise to remain at youthful levels.

The next time you see an elderly person in some state of ill repair, remember that no one would ever plan to spend their golden years bent and crippled. It's a slow process brought about by years of neglect. The miraculous benefits of regular exercise have been shown over and over again to be a virtual fountain of youth, and it's never too late to get started.

Go easy at first - adaptation occurs slowly and the only way to get anywhere is consistency. A sore body isn't necessary to make progress and will only encourage you to skip workouts. You must be willing to make exercise part of your lifestyle. There is no end and no finish line. Don't treat your fitness program as a weight loss project or you'll quit for sure. Instead, find activities you enjoy and make it a point to do something every day, even if it's only for fifteen minutes. This is how fit people think, and it's how you must think. The very act of enjoying an activity will make you better at it. The natural progression will be to learn more and, eventually, you'll be following the plan outlined for you. Every great athlete the world has ever known began as a child playing just for fun.

No one has ever started as an expert. If you've never exercised before, the world is your oyster. Your body will begin to rejuvenate as soon as you start.

"Courage is resistance to fear, mastery of fear – not absence of fear."

-Mark Twain

CHAPTER 13 - THE MIND – IT'S ALL IN YOUR HEAD

No matter how much information I give you, it's totally useless unless you put it to work. That makes this the most important chapter in the book. I wish I could just tell you to think positively, but there's much more to it than that. Let's look at what it takes to be positive.

Everything that you hear, see, feel and think is constructed by your mind. To some extent, we are all living in a dream. Based on your fears, customs, habits, intellectual abilities, and level of confidence you have already formed an imaginary picture of yourself and the world around you. What you've been taught and how you viewed your experiences help make up the person you are today. You are a product of your experiences and your own imagination. Since you have created this image, you can also change it at any time. In order to do so, you must overcome the three greatest enemies of achievement – *indecision, doubt*, and *fear.* These three travel together. Indecision causes doubt,

doubt leads to fear, and fear will stop you in your tracks. The best way to beat this unholy trio is by chipping away at them, making small changes and doing them every day. The most practical way of controlling your mind is to develop habits with a definite purpose backed by a definite plan.

ATTITUDE

A basic premise in human psychology is that most of us will make decisions based on avoiding pain and gaining pleasure, usually in that order. Anything that you associate with negatively, you will naturally move away from.

I was an example of this last summer when I traveled to Alaska to watch my brother compete in an Eco-challenge race. These races are designed to be the most physically and mentally demanding races you can run. Many of the teams don't finish, and everyone is pushed to the edge of human endurance. My brother told me he hoped we could race together some time. I unconsciously formed a picture of myself suffering even though I've never run the race before. Based on that image, I decided it wasn't something I personally wanted to do.

Quite the opposite was true for the racers. They were keyed up in anticipation. They had all spent hundreds of hours training and thousands of dollars just to be there and couldn't wait to get started. These athletes viewed the race as something very positive and fun. For them, the pain would be associated with not getting to race. When I spoke with them after four days of grueling racing they all talked about what a great experience it was. Their picture was obviously different from mine.

This is how it is for you. No matter what the challenge in life, you will enjoy only what you choose to enjoy. It's entirely up to you. If you view a healthier diet as punishment for being overweight, you won't stick with it. If you think exercise is hard work, you won't convince yourself to do it very often. You create your own reality and determine whether you're having fun or not. Imagine a picture in your mind that makes whatever you're doing a positive experience. If you want to change, reinvent yourself in your mind.

CONFIDENCE

"Knowledge is power", well almost. It becomes power only when, and if, you act on it. That's why you needed all the information you've read so far. Knowledge allows you to think for yourself. The more you learn, the more confident you become knowing the difference between positive thinking and wishful thinking.

You will be bombarded with too good to be true testimonials, miracle cures, astonishing weight loss products, and whatever else a good marketer can throw at you. Use your head to avoid the scams, because now you know better.

Make a realistic assessment of yourself and work only on being a better you. The world needs all kinds and we are all built differently. Getting caught up with impossible body images will make you lose sight of your own progress. Confidence comes from knowing where you're going and how to get there. This book was written to help show you the way.

GOAL SETTING - PERSEVERANCE

When I was thirty, I decided I wanted to learn martial arts. My goal was to get my black belt. I trained hard four to five days a week and achieved my goal in three years. During my training, I became friends with my instructor. He was a tenth degree grand master, one the highest ranked practitioners in the United States. He told me that you really only begin to learn martial arts once you've gotten your black belt and that most Americans drop out shortly after earning it. Not realizing it at the time, I followed suit and got too busy with other things not long after I earned my black belt.

What I failed to realize in the beginning is that martial arts is not a system to see how quickly you can learn certain movements and advance to the next level. It's a lifestyle that you can take with you into old age. I have seen clumsy, overweight women become graceful and break boards. Remarkably, this change happened for virtually everyone, some faster and more easily than others, but everyone progressed if they continued to show up. Today, I am probably not much better at martial arts than when I began, even though I achieved my goal. Because my original goal was faulty, I failed to grasp the big picture and missed the most important lesson - perseverance.

If your goal is to lose 20 pounds in 3 months, you can probably do it. You can count every calorie and work out like you're going to the Olympics, but once you achieve your goal, like most people, you will lose interest and slowly go back to your old ways. Of course, you'll put the weight back on and be no better off than when you started. The weight loss industry caters to America's need for immediate gratification and goal setting. Lifestyle changes are different. You have to make them part of you. It's easy to do if you take your time, and get over your fears. Get on a good program, keep showing up, and you'll progress at your own pace. How can you lose?

ELIMINATE FEAR

Fear is probably the most negative of all human emotions. It doesn't exist in any object or situation; your fears are totally constructed in your mind. You may have been taught your fears by others, or formed them based on past failures or weaknesses, but they're not real. They are your own personal creation, designed to control your behavior. Your fears exist in your subconscious mind, and they will be real to you until you identify them and work to eliminate them. The following are a few of the most common reasons people don't take action.

Fear of failure has crept into everyone's mind at one time or another. It's the fear that we may not have what it takes. Giving into this fear gives you an excuse to quit. It's a self-fulfilling prophecy that keeps you from finding out what you're capable of. If you get that feeling that you might not be able to do something or will somehow embarrass yourself, do it anyway. The only way to fail is to give up, or, worse yet, not even try. The shame you fear is a figment of your imagination. By visualizing success rather than failure, believing 'I can do it' rather than 'I can't', you prevent your own negative thoughts from taking control of you. I don't know why we choose to ignore the ninety-nine "that a boys" to hear the one "you're not good enough."

Fear of change keeps you in a rut. You probably have no idea how most of your daily habits began. Whether you're aware of it or not, your daily routine has been chosen by you. Most of our habits have crept into our daily lives without any thought; yet it's amazing how people will vehemently defend their routine because they fear change will be uncomfortable. No growth can occur without change. Whether in your mind, or in the gym, it's the process of adapting to new stimulus that causes growth. Embrace the changes in your life. Know that even if there is some discomfort, you are growing stronger from the experience.

Fear of success is a fear that's hard to accept because everyone believes that they want to be successful. This fear will cause you to unconsciously sabotage your progress. It comes into play when you believe that you are unworthy of success, and will lose something by being successful. Ironically, most often it's the fear of losing our excuses. They are road blocks you've accidentally put up yourself. If you carry the beliefs that fit people are vain, thin women are snobby, rich people are greedy, or whatever else comes to mind, they're the defenses you've put up for your own short comings. Don't sell yourself short by falling in love with your potential, thinking you could do it if you wanted to, but never taking that step to find out. If you find you carry a negative belief about yourself or someone else, replace it with a positive one. Self-improvement is only for you, and your success should only be measured by you.

Be diligent to find out what's stopping you. Health and happiness are not goals in life, but states of mind. It's a spiritual journey that everyone must take alone. God has given you the free will to choose whether your mental attitude is your most valuable asset or your worst enemy. History has shown that we can do anything we put our minds to. The same powers that built the pyramids and sent a man to the moon are within you. Getting into shape shouldn't be too tough.

TAKE ACTION

Nike® said it best - Just do it! When you act on a thought with emotion and faith you are taking part in the process of creation. This formula has been the model of achievement throughout history and is the even in the Bible. Jesus taught that with enough faith you can move mountains, but that faith is useless without action. Faith overcomes fear and develops perseverance. These are the lessons behind miracle-making, and you can apply them to any situation. When you erase all doubt, anything is possible, but you still have to move. Adopt the mindset that you are responsible for all that you are or are not, and look to yourself as the cause and solution to all your problems. The actions you have taken up till now have been in the process of creating what you are at this very moment whether you choose to acknowledge it or not. Stop right now and decide to put the past behind you. Find the positive in every situation and then go for it and live your dreams. You'll find that miraculously you will get all the help you need.

Just as you're probably not going to win the lottery to pay your debts, you're not going to get out of an unhealthy lifestyle by luck either. You need to make a decision, have faith, and act on that decision. The more often you can do this the more powerful you will become.

Reading this book has raised your awareness. Use that knowledge to take new actions and you will end up at a different place. By putting your new thoughts into motion everyday, they will eventually become automatic and take on a life of their own. That's why you can't miss a single day at first.

The only time you can be certain of is right now, so live for today. Decide you will enjoy the process, believe in what you're doing, stick with it, and don't give that little voice the chance to talk you out of it. Decide today to better yourself and **"JUST DO IT!"**

You have absolute control over only one thing and that is your thoughts. If you fail to control your own mind, you can be sure you will control nothing else. You must learn to protect your mind from the poisons of negative suggestions and fill it with positive thoughts and love for others. This is how you feed the most powerful force you possess - your spirit.

"In the middle of difficulty lies opportunity."

-Albert Einstein

CHAPTER 14 - TIME TO GET STARTED

PHASE I

If you've never exercised before or are very overweight, start at Phase I. The goal is to slowly change your daily routine and build up your nutritional status. Just take it one day at a time and don't quit. If you suffer a set back, start again, the good days will add up, you'll see. If you already exercise on a regular basis, focus strictly on the nutritional portion of phase I and move on to phase II.

You must start by supplementing with all the essential nutrients. Everything from your mood to your waistline is dependent on it. You simply cannot get what you need from food today. If you do nothing else, proper nutritional supplementation will afford you some protection. Don't throw away healthy years of living by thinking otherwise. **NUTRALL** was designed specifically for this purpose; it makes it easy to get it right and covers every nutrient in this book. You can read more about **NUTRALL** in the back of the book.

MONTH ONE a) Replace one meal with a **NUTRALL** shake, preferably breakfast. This is one of the most important steps. Building up your nutritional status will help control your cravings, increase your energy level, and remind you everyday to change your old habits.

b) Eliminate sweet drinks (soft drinks, fruit juices, sweetened teas) and drink water.

c) Walk briskly for 15 minutes every day.

MONTH TWO a) Do same steps as above.

b) Eat a light mid-morning snack. Use only whole foods.

c) Extend walk to 30 minutes six days a week.

The purpose of your daily walks is not to melt off the pounds, it won't. It's to help you develop an exercise schedule, and boost your metabolism. Try to do your exercise at the same time every day, preferably in the morning. It will make it much easier to form a habit. Don't do anything to make it more difficult, just leave your house and walk briskly in one direction for 8-15 minutes and turn around and walk back. Keep track of the date you started so you will continue to move on with the program. Be aware that walking will not build a beautiful body. Form follows function, and your body will conform to how you train it. That's why sprinters look different than marathon runners, and people who work out with weights look different than people who just do aerobic exercise. It's the time, not the activity, that's important right now. This is time you're making for yourself. Make sure you enjoy every minute of it. Use the time to clear your mind of internal chatter or negative thoughts, and project in your mind a positive image of how you want your body and your life to be. Then, behave as though you are already there.

Eat raw fruit or vegetables with a small amount of protein for your mid morning snack. You'll probably have to pack some food when for you're at work, so plan ahead. Small portions of chicken or turkey and an apple or cucumber are good cold. Be creative with foods you like. You're not eating a meal here so don't think too hard about finding the perfect food. Just make sure you eat something healthy between breakfast and lunch. Low fat yogurt will do in a pinch.

MONTH THREE   a) Do the same steps as in Months One and Two.

b) Add some simple stretches after your walk.

(See Appendix.)

c) Whenever possible, replace starches like breads, potatoes, white rice, and pasta, with vegetables.

Add some intermittent jogging on days that you feel good. Don't over do it, you don't need to be sore to make progress. Be militant about not missing any days.

They don't all have to be good workouts, just keep showing up.

MONTH FOUR

Congratulations! If you've made it this far you have developed the habits you need to go the distance and are well on your way to having the fitness and body you want. You will never have to spend more time than this on your body.

Now use the fitness time you've created on other activities: yoga, martial arts, pilates, dance, whatever suits you. Make sure you find something that interests you. This is a very important next step to avoid boredom. The collective consciousness of group activities will also boost your energy and help keep you motivated. These types of activities are usually 1-3 days per week, so continue your regular routine on the other days.

PHASE II

Your exercise schedule should be routine now. Your next task should be an effort towards eliminating the negative aspects of your eating habits. This doesn't mean you can never eat any of these foods, although it would be nice. It's the habitual consumption of altered foods that will eventually bring you down.

FIRST: Eliminate free radicals from altered fats. Start with these:

- Refined vegetable oils, and frozen desserts

- Salad dressings. Use vinegar and spices with some extra virgin olive oil
- Deep fried foods (heated polyunsaturated oils are killers)
- Margarine (use butter)

SECOND: Eliminate sugar. This step alone will have remarkable effects. Not only will you shed unwanted pounds, your thinking will be clearer, your mood will improve, and you will be less sore. Look for these culprits in your diet.

- Colas or soft drinks, this includes diet drinks (drink water)
- Fruit juice (the fresh fruit is fine)
- Honey
- Table sugar
- Corn syrup
- Candy
- Ice cream
- Pastries
- Boxed or bagged cereals

Giving up sugar is not easy, and you don't have to do it all at once. If you get a craving, go for raw fruit before you give in, plan ahead so you'll have some around. Take this step seriously, all this sugar is surely making you fat and sick.

You can stay at this level for as long as you like, but your body will eventually adapt to the exercise and you won't make any new progress.

TIME TO JOIN THE GYM

Now, get ready to build some muscle if you really want to change your body. Aerobic exercise alone won't do it. For long-term success your focus must be on building muscle. Muscle supports your skeleton, provides amino acids for your immune system, and gives the shape to your figure. Muscle is where we burn bodyfat!

There are other advantages to resistance exercise that are not as obvious. When you lift weights, you signal your body to adapt to the stress by making your muscles, tendons, ligaments and bones stronger. In response, you secrete higher levels of growth hormone and testosterone, which, in turn, encourages the formation of lean tissue and the reduction of bodyfat. These are the same hormones used by expensive anti-aging clinics. They don't work without the exercise anyway, so it's better to just make your own.

Don't be intimidated by lifting weights. It's easy to learn and you'll feel fantastic when you've finished. Weight training programs are beyond the scope of this book. I recommend you hire a personal trainer for a few sessions to show you the basics and to make sure you're doing the exercises correctly. You can also pick up one of the many beginning weight-training books from your local library or bookstore. Keep your weight workouts under an hour. Sports science has shown that any longer will diminish your results.

PHASE III

If you choose to continue your sport at a competitive level, don't guess on your training. You are an athlete now and you need to start thinking like one. If you haven't done so already, seek out a coach to take you to the next level of your sport. I highly recommend that you read *The New Power Program* by Dr. Michael Colgan. The information there is indispensable to all athletes.

BOTTOM LINE

If you've been exercising and not making progress, your diet is probably to blame. Exercise increases your body's needs for nutrients. Without them, exercising puts an additional load on an already malnourished system. Don't start without a complete nutritional supplement that assures sufficient amounts of vitamins, minerals, essential fats, and protein.

Unless your body is adequately nourished, you will forever be fighting a losing battle with fat. Malnutrition is the main reason most people get fat in the first place. Without sufficient nutrition, you will never be able to stop over eating, exercise loses its benefits, and your health will ultimately suffer.

Be patient. Tissue changes occur slowly but surely. Changes in your appearance may feel like they're taking an eternity, but change you will. You probably didn't notice yourself getting fatter from day to day either. It's better to learn to love the process and the power that comes from challenging yourself. You will feel the reward in your soul when you care for, and utilize, your most valuable asset.

> *"I asked for all things that I might enjoy life.*
> *I was given life that I might enjoy all things."*
>
> *unknown*

If you aren't able to find the time to exercise (about 15 - 45 minutes) you've found part of your problem and should give this book to someone who can use it. There's simply no reward for a sedentary lifestyle.

"It is one of the most beautiful compensations of this life that no man can sincerely try to help another without helping himself."

-Emerson

CONCLUSION

This whole project began many years ago. It began quietly and out of necessity. I had severe degenerative arthritis in my ankle and because I was unwilling to accept my disability, I found the answers I was looking for. In writing this book, I'm hoping to pass some of those lessons along to you. I became a chiropractor because of that ankle and, now, an author. As I sit here nearing the end of this project, I am pain free and wondering what opportunities will come your way because of what you once perceived as a disability.

I presume you've read this book because you're looking for answers. To the best of my abilities, I have given you the truth, even if it's not what you wanted to hear. The truth can be that way sometimes. Use the information because it works. It's a common sense approach to your health and waistline, based on medical and nutritional science. Stick with the program and, eventually, it's going to be just as automatic to do the right things as your old destructive habits were. You don't need to become a sociopath counting calories, quit your job and learn to cook, or spend your life shopping for special foods. If some of the recommendations seem too strict, remember that they are the ideals. Don't make yourself crazy trying to be perfect. None of us are. Just keep making little changes, and you'll get there.

Modern science will not out smart nature, so don't immediately look to drugs for answers to your physical and mental problems. Most of the health problems you will encounter in your lifetime will, in some way, be a result of poor nutrition. Now you're in possession of enough information to start doing something about it.

Make this the beginning of new learning. Your body and the spirit that resides in it are all that you really have in this world, don't neglect either one. Just as your body eventually becomes what you eat, so your spirit is fed by what you put in your mind. Put only good things into both. Learn to meditate, read books on positive thinking, try new exercises, take up a new sport, and pass your new knowledge on to your children. Life will give you whatever you ask from it.

Be fearless in your pursuit. Know without doubt that you can do what you put your mind to and avoid anyone who belittles your efforts. Only a failure, trying to justify their own mediocrity, would depreciate anyone's plan to better themselves. Share your plans with those who support you, and keep them to yourself around those that don't.

Finally, what will you do without your health? Where will you go to find pleasure? Your physical attractiveness, ability to enjoy a sunset, play with your children, enjoy sex, travel, everything we take for granted relies on good health. If you lose it, you would surely give up all that you have to get it back. Don't take this gift for granted. Your health in the future will be a result of the investment you make today.

Now, it's up to you. The government won't help you, science can't save you, and our health care practitioners are trapped in a system that makes no profit from keeping you well. We live in a culture that has sold everyone on convenience and immediate gratification, and you've been paying the price for it with your health.

Ultimately, you will decide the true measure of your success. By thinking only in terms of self-improvement you enter an arena where you always win. If, in these pages, you found the answers you'd been looking for, I encourage you to take action. Invest in yourself. I can think of no better place to spend your time or money.

If you have questions or think you would benefit from coaching, you can reach me at **www.theeatinggame.com**.

APPENDIX:

POPULAR WEIGHT LOSS TRENDS

HIGH PROTEIN, LOW CARBOHYDRATE DIETS

Carbohydrates and insulin has become the red-headed stepchild of many popular diet programs. Atkins, Protein Power, and the like recommend high protein, high fat diets with little or no carbohydrate in order to reduce insulin levels. These diets promise the loss of pounds and inches and they work at first.
Fat is digested slower and suppresses your appetite longer than carbohydrates. Since refined carbohydrates are a large part of the diet of most overweight people, when you eliminate them, your total calorie intake is usually greatly reduced. In many cases, you simply have a low calorie diet. You also lose a lot of water on a high protein diet, which gives the illusion of weight loss. For a few people this may be the best way to eat, but, for most, these diets offer yet another short term fix to this countries blubber battle.

This strategy also carries numerous detrimental side effects when combined with the problems in our modern food supply, first and foremost are nutritional deficiencies. These diets are seriously deficient in vitamins and minerals and expose you to high levels of harmful fat and chemicals. The Eskimos, who are always used as examples for these programs because they remain healthy on high fat, high protein diets, eat wild game and fish that have harvested the rich nutrients from the sea. Those nutrients are in the flesh of those animals. The thought that there can be any comparison to our modern day food supply is nothing short of ridiculous. Maybe the worst part of these high protein low carbohydrate diet plans is that they prime you to put on *more* fat should you ever go back to your original eating habits.

The truth is that insulin metabolism is dependant on many nutritional factors and even other hormones. It's been demonstrated that with proper nutrition, laboratory animals don't develop insulin disorders, even when fed a diet that would normally cause diabetes. If you insist on making the least possible effort, these programs may be a reasonable intervention, but be sure you supplement. You would be much better off avoiding such fanaticism, in time it will only leave you sore, weak and tired. As I wrote this chapter Dr. Atkins suffered a heart attack.

FAT BURNING FORMULAS

Most thermogenic or fat burning formulas rely on a combination of caffeine, ephedrine, and aspirin as their active ingredients. This combination slows down the time it takes for your body to accommodate to the stimulants caffeine and ephedrine. Stimulants reduce your appetite and raise your metabolism. However, the effects are only temporary and, like all drugs, you will need to keep increasing the dosage to get the same effects. Then when you quit, you will of course, quickly rebound back to your old fat level, plus a little more. Drugs are never going to be the answer.

CARBOHYDRATE AND FAT BLOCKERS

These products do interfere with the absorption of dietary carbohydrates and fats. The problem is that you're supposed to absorb them. When they are left to putrefy in your digestive tract, you expose yourself to high levels of toxic by-products and your fellow man to some pretty bad gas. This type of intervention only encourages you to continue to eat poorly, which is the problem in the first place.

TAKING A SECOND STEP WITH DIFFICULT CONDITIONS

The information presented here is useful for difficult conditions where the cause is unknown. This second step has proven effective in improving symptoms that haven't responded to the changes you've already made. Examples are allergies, chronic fatigue syndrome, fibromyalgia, migraine headaches, colitis, autoimmune diseases, and many others.

This extra step is only necessary if you don't improve on the regular program. It's aimed at removing allergenic foods from your diet. It's pretty simple stuff, but you should still always consult with your doctor.

LEAKY GUT SYNDROME

Leaky Gut Syndrome (LGS) is a poorly recognized, but common, health disorder. The basic lesion is an intestinal lining that is more permeable than normal. It's caused by *inflammation of the gut lining* that results in abnormally large spaces between the cells that line the digestive tract. This condition allows toxic material to enter the blood stream that would otherwise be repelled and eliminated, including undigested proteins and fats.

Under normal circumstances your body is only exposed to tiny food antigens (proteins). When large food antigens get through, as is the case with LGS, your body's defenses are activated as they would be against an intruder. When your body produces antibodies against once harmless and innocuous food, you have a food allergy. Every time you eat the offending food, you aggravate your symptoms.

The inflammation also damages the carrier proteins in your digestive tract. They normally work like little revolving doors to transport nutrients from your intestinal tract to your blood stream, so this syndrome can lead to a long list of vitamin and mineral deficiencies. Nutritional deficiencies, of course, weaken your body and can alter your immune responses.

In theory, a malfunctioning immune system may produce antibodies against your body's own tissue if they are similar to the offending antigen. This is a plausible theory for the formation of autoimmune diseases.

Inflammation of the gut lining can be brought about by the following:

- High refined carbohydrate diet. (re-read section on sugar)
- Chemicals in processed foods (dyes, preservatives, peroxidised fats)
- Over use of alcohol and caffeine (strong gut irritants)
- Enzyme deficiencies (e.g. intolerance to gluten containing foods),
- Lactose intolerance, (inability to digest dairy).
- Antibiotics, because they kill both harmful and beneficial bacteria, they can lead to overgrowth of harmful organisms in the gastrointestinal tract.
- Over use of non-steroidal anti-inflammatory drugs (aspirin, ibuprofen, etc.)
- Prescription corticosteroids (e.g. prednisone)
- Food and beverages contaminated by bacteria or parasites.
- Prolonged stress

HOW TO REVERSE THE LEAKY GUT SYNDROME

The intestinal lining must be allowed to heal. This requires the nutritional support we have already talked about, and removal of the foods most likely to cause allergies.

GUIDELINES FOR HYPOALLERGENIC FOODS

1.) Eliminate all dairy products, including milk, cheese, cream, cottage cheese, yogurt, butter, frozen yogurt, and ice cream. Avoid any products made with casein (a milk protein)

2.) Eliminate fatty meats like beef, pork, and veal. Acceptable choices are chicken, turkey, lamb, and fish. Choose free range or organic products whenever they are available. Also watch how you cook them. Deep frying is not acceptable.

3.) Eliminate gluten. Avoid foods that contain wheat, oat, rye, barley, and malt. Common foods containing gluten are breads, cereal, pasta, crackers, and any product made with flour containing these grains. Acceptable choices are rice, millet, potato, tapioca, and gluten free flour. This is the most difficult part of the diet, but also the most important.

4.) Avoid alcohol - beer, wine, liquor, and products that contain alcohol.

5.) Avoid caffeine - coffee, teas, soda pop, and thermogenic supplements.

6.) Avoid processed foods - refined sugar, refined carbohydrates, peanuts, cheese, and vinegar

7.) Drink at least two quarts of water per day.

Stay with the diet for at least two weeks or longer until symptoms subside. As you have already learned it takes some gusto to make big food changes, even for this short period of time, but, I assure you it is well worth it. Additional nutritional support beyond your existing program may be required to aid in the process of rebuilding healthier cells.

HYPOALLERGENIC FOOD LIST		
FOOD GROUP	**EAT**	**DON'T EAT**
MEAT, FISH, POULTRY	CHICKEN, TURKEY. LAMB	RED MEAT. COLD CUTS
LEGUMES, EGGS	COLD WATER FISH, SALMON HALIBUT, TROUT, LEGUMES	SAUSAGE, HOT DOGS, EGGS
DAIRY PRODUCTS	MILK SUBSTITUTES, RICE MILK SOY MILK, NUT MILKS	MILK, CHEESE, COTTAGE CHEESE. YOGURT, ICE CREAM, CREAM
STARCH	WHITE OR SWEET POTATO, RICE TATAPIOCA, BUCKWHEAT. MILLET	CORN, OR CORN CONTAIMNG PRODUCTS, PASTA
BREAD CEREAL	ANY MADE FROM RICE, MILLET BUCKWHEAT, SOY. QUINOA POTATO FLOUR, GLUTEN FREE FLOUR BASED PRODUCTS. SPELT	ANYTHING MADE WITH WHEAT. OAT, RYE, BARLEY
VEGETABLES	ALL VEGETABLES, FRESH OR FROZEN ARE BEST	CREAMED VEGETABLES OR PROHIBITED INGREDIENTS
FRUITS	ALL, EXCEPT CITRUS AND STRAWBERRIES, BEST FRESH OR FROZEN	FRUIT DRINKS, ADES, CITRUS, STRAWBERRIES
BEVERAGES	WATER, UNSWEETENED FRUIT OR VEGETABLE JUICE, HERBAL TEA	MILK, COFFE, TEA, SODA POP CITRUS DRINKS. COCKTAILS
FATS / OILS	NUTRALL ESSENTIAL OILS, OLIVE OIL. SESAME	MARGERINE, SHORTENING, BUTTER, SALAD DRESSING DEEP FRYING
SOUP	VEGETABLE BASED BROTH, CHILE MADE WITH GROUND CHICKEN OR TURKEY	CANNED OR CREAMED

This should be enough to get you started. The idea is to let your body detoxify and heal. Once this is accomplished, you can add certain foods back into your diet if they don't cause symptoms. Having fun is a big part of being healthy, so make the effort to build up your resistance so you don't have to needlessly suffer.

WHAT IS NUTRALL?

WWW.NUTRALL.COM

NUTRALL is a potent blend of concentrated whey protein, essential fats, carbohydrate, vitamins, minerals, trace elements, and dietary fiber. Originally created to meet the higher nutritional demands of athletes and people suffering with chronic diseases, **NUTRALL** provides the nutritional base needed to start any program.

The development of **NUTRALL** came about out of necessity as most tools do. There was no easy way for me to make the over sixty essential nutrients available to patients. One trip to the health food store with the information that you have now will drive that point home. The nutrients you ingest must also be accompanied by the right amounts of protein, carbohydrate and essential fats to work properly in your body. It was clear that a specific product would have to be formulated to provide you all your nutrients.

NUTRALL is a true meal replacement, not a supplement. For about the cost of a fast food burger or a latte, you can eat something that will actually do you some good. Because **NUTRALL** is to be taken in place of a meal that you would have eaten anyway, it costs you nothing.

I recommend taking **NUTRALL** in the morning in order to help eliminate the refined carbohydrates that most people consume for breakfast in the form of boxed cereals, pastries, bagels, and the like. This will also help you make better food choices throughout the day by satisfying your nutrient cravings. However, you can replace any meal you like.

It can be difficult to get your metabolism back to normal once you've drained your nutrient reserves with dieting and junk food. In order to overcome a deficiency, you have to consume many times the U.S. recommended daily allowance to rebuild your nutrient stores. It won't happen without careful nutritional supplementation. **NUTRALL** is a good place to start and, though this process takes time, you'll feel the difference in just a couple of weeks.

The real answer for most of you is so beautifully simple that this book could have been only one page long. Replace the nutrients that have been lost from our modern food supply and avoid the foods that drain your body. Basically if you supplement correctly, and stick to whole foods, meats, vegetables, and fruits you will be way ahead of the game. Hundreds of thousands of years of evolution can't be wrong and your body will start working for you instead of against you. It's ridiculously easy, and unbelievably effective. If you're willing to spend thirty seconds a day to turn on your blender and stick with it, you'll be well on your way to having the body and health you want.

INGREDIENTS

NUTRALL is formulated to represent the most absorbable and biologically active forms of vitamins and minerals. A plant-derived colloidal mineral supplement provides the trace minerals normally found in topsoil, and is nearly 100% absorbable. **NUTRALL** contains a high quality whey protein concentrate, and a special blend of cold pressed organic seed oils. The final ratio is 40-30-30 carbohydrate, protein and essential fat. **NUTRALL** is sweetened with fructose. This natural fruit sugar doesn't have the same negative effects as glucose because it has to pass through the liver before it can be utilized. **NUTRALL** contains no artificial sweeteners.

Each serving of **NUTRALL** contains:

Whey protein	36g
Essential fatty acids	14g
Complex carbohydrate	47g
Dietary fiber	8g

also contains:

Vitamin A	150%	Folic acid	100%	Chromium	160%
Beta Carotene	5000 IU	Biotin	50%	Selenium	140%
Vitamin C	800%	Vitamin K	100%	Manganese	100%
Biofalvinoids	50mg	Choline	25mg	Molybdenum	67%
Vitamin E	600%	Inositol	25mg	Copper	1mg
VitaminD	50%	PABA	12.5mg	Boron	1mg
VitaminB1	300%	CoQ10	5mg	Potassium	700mg
Vitamin B2	300%	Pycnogenol	20mg	Sodium	72mg
VitaminB3	125%	Calcium	500mg	Bromelain	20mg
VitaminB5	180%	Magnesium	250mg	Lactase	5mg
VitaminB6	250%	Silica	100mg	*and also contains a complete range of trace minerals*	
VitaminB12	400%	Zinc	100%		

"There is hardly anything in this world, that some man cannot make a little worse and sell a little cheaper, and the people who consider price only are this man's lawful prey."
-John Ruskin

VITAMINS

Vitamin B1 - **(Thiamin)** is involved in energy metabolism. Symptoms associated with thiamin deficiency are congestive heart failure (Beriberi), memory loss, depression, weakness, paralysis, emotional instability, and loss of appetite. The best sources of thiamin are whole grains. Up to 100 percent of thiamin is lost in processing and baking.

Vitamin B2 - **(Riboflavin)** is involved in energy production by the mitochondria inside your cells. Meat, poultry, and fish are good sources. Food processing can destroy up to 80 percent. Riboflavin deficiency is characterized by soreness and burning of the lips, mouth and tongue, light sensitivity, inflammation at the corners of the mouth, anemia, and neuropathy.

Vitamin B3 - **(Niacin)** functions in energy production and cellular respiration. Niacin deficiency (Pellagra) is marked by dermatitis on exposed parts of the body, mental disturbances, and diarrhea. The best food sources are meat and fish.

Vitamin B5 - **(Pantothenic acid)** is involved in energy production. It is also essential for making steroid hormones (testosterone, estrogen) and brain neurotransmitters. Signs of deficiency include; "burning feet," depression, and disturbed sleep.

Vitamin B6 - **(Pyridoxine)** functions in energy production and is vital to protein and amino acid metabolism. Good food sources are chicken, fish, and eggs. Vitamin B6 is involved in the conversion of the amino acid tryptophan to niacin, so a B6 deficiency produces many of the same symptoms. Oral contraceptives interfere with the utilization of B6, as do other drugs.

Vitamin B12 - (Cyanocobalamin) is required for the maturation of red blood cells and is part of coenzymes found in all cells, particularly rapid- turnover cells. Deficiency produces (Pernicious anemia) damaging your nerves and spinal cord. Left untreated, pernicious anemia leads to insanity and eventual death. **Animal foods are the only sources of B12, so unsupplemented vegetarians are likely to be deficient.**

Folic Acid - is involved in amino acid metabolism, especially rapid-turnover cells. High doses of folic acid can mask a B12 deficiency. The best sources are dark green leafy vegetables and egg yolks. Folic acid deficiency is widespread in the U.S. and is directly associated with birth defects (spina bifida), other symptoms include anemia, and poor growth of new cells.

Biotin - is essential for making glucose and fats available for fuel. Biotin is also involved in the breaking down and building up of new proteins. Symptoms of biotin deficiency are eczema, baldness, depression, gray hair, and increased pain sensitivity.

Some biotin is made in your digestive tract by friendly bacteria. Food sources are egg yolks and liver.

Vitamin C (Ascorbic acid) is used by your body in the formation of collagen, the connective tissue that holds your body together. It is also an anti-oxidant that protects your cells from the negative effects of oxidation. Vitamin C is involved in folic acid metabolism and bone formation. A deficiency causes *scurvy*, a disease of collagen break down and is characterized by bleeding tendency (bleeding gums, easy and excessive bruising), and poor wound healing. Other vitamin C deficiency symptoms are weight loss, high risk for infection, loose teeth, increased cancer risk, and swollen joints. It takes only a small amount of vitamin C each day to prevent scurvy, but much more for optimum health. Adequate vitamin C is required for the release of growth hormone and many other bodily functions. Make sure you get enough!

Bioflavonoids - Compounds linked to the functions of vitamin C. Research suggests bioflavonoids may have anti-aging and anti-cancer properties.

Vitamin E - (d-alpha-tocopherol) is a fat soluble vitamin that mainly functions as an anti-oxidant. Vitamin E protects essential and unsaturated fats from oxidation (keeps fats from going rancid inside our body). Deficiency causes age spots, lowered immunity, weakness, and muscle pain. Vitamin E deficiency has been implicated in Alzheimer's Syndrome, and increased cancer risk. Vitamin C recharges spent vitamin E so it can be reused.

Vitamin A - (Retinol) is a fat soluble vitamin that is essential for vision, reproduction, cell growth, immune function, maintenance of skin and mucus membranes, and has possible roles in steroid hormone formation and hemoglobin synthesis. Symptoms of vitamin A deficiency are; night blindness, infertility, birth defects, weakened immune system, poor growth, acne, and increased cancer risk.

Vitamin A can be toxic if taken in excess of 25,000 lUs/ day over time.

Beta- carotene can be converted to vitamin A by your body and serves as an anti-oxidant independent of its vitamin A functions. Beta-carotene is non-toxic, but may turn your skin orange if taken in very large amounts.

Vitamin D - (Cholecalciferol) is a fat soluble vitamin closely involved with calcium and phosphorus metabolism. It is essential for bone growth and mineral balance in the body. Your body makes Vitamin D when your skin is exposed to sunlight. Dependence on dietary sources of vitamin D varies with climate and influences that restrict sunlight.

Vitamin D deficiency causes (Rickets) or soft bones caused by poor mineralization that can produce skeletal deformities in children. Other symptoms are bone pain, muscle weakness, and arthritis. It's unlikely that you're deficient on a reasonable diet, and high doses of vitamin D can be toxic.

Vitamin K - (Phylloquinone) is a fat-soluble vitamin essential for blood clotting.

Choline - can be made by your body, but the majority still comes from the diet.

Choline forms neurotransmitters in your brain and is involved in memory. It is an essential component of every cell membrane. Choline also has functions in energy production. Choline deficiency may have involvement in Alzheimer's disease.

Inositol - is also made by the body and found in food. Inositol is essential for insulin and calcium metabolism.

Coenzyme Q10 - can be made by the body and is found in food. It is essential for energy production in every cell, and is also a powerful anti-oxidant. CoQ10 is involved in the maintenance of your immune system and has been shown to have anti-viral and antibacterial activity. Incidence of CoQ10 deficiency increases with age.

Pycnogenol - (grape seed extract) is a potent anti-oxidant that crosses the blood brain barrier to help protect brain and nerve tissue.

MINERALS

Ag - Silver is believed to be an essential element, not because it is required for an enzyme system, but as a systemic disinfectant and immune system support. Silver is an anti-bacterial, anti-viral, and anti-fungal metabolite that disables specific enzymes that micro-organisms use for respiration. Silver deficiency results in an impaired immune system.

Al - Aluminum is found in high concentrations in all plants, including food crops. You cannot eat any grain, vegetable, fruit, nut, or drink any natural water source without taking in large quantities of aluminum. Aluminum's known biological function is to activate the enzyme succinic dehydrogenase. The aluminum found in plants is organically-bound colloidal aluminum and does not appear to have any negative effect. In fact, it is essential to human nutrition. The aluminum believed to be implicated in Alzheimer's Disease is linked to chronic exposure to metallic aluminum from industrial pollutants. These studies may prove to be flawed anyway, as other studies show that deficiencies of other nutrients may be responsible for this degenerative brain disease.

As - Arsenic functions in enzyme systems. Arsenic metabolism is affected by zinc, selenium, arginine, choline, methionine, and taurine. Metallic arsenic is 65 times more toxic than organically bound arsenic. Arsenic deficiency may be involved in carpal tunnel syndrome, TMJ, and repetitive motion type degeneration.

Au - Gold has been reported to be helpful against joint inflammation, but is not usually effective in advanced rheumatoid arthritis. Gold may have anti-inflammatory effects but can also have toxic reactions when used at therapeutic dosages.

B - Boron is essential for bone metabolism and efficient use of calcium and magnesium. Boron is also required for normal levels of the sex hormones testosterone and estrogen.

C - Carbon is the essential structural atom for all organic molecules. Carbohydrates, proteins, fats, vitamins, and enzymes, all have a carbon skeletons.

Ca - Calcium is the most abundant mineral in the human body. Ninety-nine percent of calcium is stored in bones and teeth. The other 1% is involved in nerve conduction and muscle contractions as well as other vital functions such as blood clotting, the release of neurotransmitters, and metabolic effects on hormones and enzymes. Calcium deficiency is common and is aggravated by other nutrients that are rich in the American diet.

Calcium is another example of the delicate balanced interactions of our food. For example, diets that are high in salt and protein increase calcium excretion. However, salt restricted diets result in decreased stomach acid causing low calcium absorption. It has been demonstrated that salt sensitivity resulting in essential hypertension can be attributed to restricted calcium and potassium intake, not elevated salt.

Calcium deficiency is further complicated by deficiencies of magnesium, boron, copper, sulfur, selenium, actinium, fluoride, strontium and or excesses of phosphorus (soft drinks), fluoride (tap water), cadmium (cigarettes), and fat. Common symptoms associated with calcium deficiencies are osteoporosis, arthritis, high blood pressure, bone spurs, muscle cramps and twitches, low back pain, kidney stones and insomnia.

CI - Chloride works with sodium and potassium to regulate fluid and electrolyte balance. Chloride is also the basic raw material our bodies use to make stomach acid (HCL). Sodium chloride (salt) is the universal source of chloride ions.

Co - Cobalt is the central atom of vitamin B12. B12 is absorbed only in the presence of intrinsic factor which is secreted by the stomach. Deficiency causes the serious disease pernicious anemia, resulting in demylination of the spinal cord, blindness, insanity and eventually death.. The only sources of B 12 are animal foods, so unsupplemented vegetarians are most likely to be deficient. Others at risk are those with malabsorption diseases (allergies to wheat gluten, cow's milk, albumen, etc.) Hypochlorhydria (low stomach acid) from a salt deficiency or heavy antacid use can affect B12 absorption. Also at risk are people who have had surgical removal of parts of the stomach (loss of intrinsic factor).

Cr - Chromium is essential for glucose metabolism, insulin metabolism, protein metabolism, and fatty acid metabolism. Food processing removes up to 90% of this important mineral. Diseases associated with chromium deficiency are diabetes, hypoglycemia, hyperinsulinism, ADD/ADHD, depression, negative nitrogen balance (protein loss), high cholesterol, elevated triglycerides, and coronary artery disease. It's been estimated that 90% of Americans are chromium deficient. Chromium deficiency is complicated by vanadium deficiency. The supplemental form, chromium picolinate, has been shown to be effective in increasing muscle mass and reducing body fat. It is the form of chromium you should use.

Cs - Cesium behaves similarly to sodium and potassium. Cesium participates in ion antagonism with potassium. Cesium chloride has been used in alternative cancer therapies.

Cu - Copper is an essential co-factor for hundreds of enzymes. Copper is involved in the functions of RNA and DNA, hair and skin pigmentation, the tensile strength of elastic fibers in blood vessels, skin, vertebral discs, and many others. Copper deficiency is widespread, though it is difficult to measure. Some symptoms associated with copper deficiency are white hair, gray hair, dry brittle hair, sagging skin (breasts, eye lids, stomach, etc.), hernias, varicose veins, aneurysms, arthritis, and ruptured vertebral discs.

F - Fluorine is an essential mineral that has shown apparent benefit to tooth enamel in reducing dental caries (cavities). The fluoridation of drinking water is still highly controversial. Fluoride toxicity appears as mottling of teeth in children. A 1990 study done by the U.S Public Health Service showed an increase in certain cancers in animal studies.

Fe - Iron functions mainly as the oxygen carrying red pigment in your blood (hemoglobin). Although iron is widely available in food many people are still deficient. "Pica" is a specific sign of iron deficiency and is characterized in adults and children who eat ice, dirt or lead paint. Symptoms of iron deficiency are anemia, fatigue, heart palpitations on exertion, and reduced cognition. *Never take iron supplements by themselves, iron can be very toxic and excess iron is difficult for the body to get rid of. Excess iron can increase your risk for bacterial infection, oxidative damage, and increases the need for selenium, copper, zinc, etc.*

Ga - Gallium has specific enzyme activity in the human brain.

Ge - Germanium is known to enhance the immune system. Many healing herbs contain relatively high levels of germanium. Deficiencies of germanium are characterized by severely reduced immune status, arthritis, low energy, and cancer.

Hg - Mercury has long been known to be a toxic element. Major sources of mercury contamination are paint, dental amalgams, pharmaceutical drugs, agricultural fungicides, and the burning of fossil fuels. There is a metabolic antagonism between mercury and selenium. The presence of selenium provides protection against mercury poisoning.

I - Iodine is required to make your thyroid hormones which control your energy. Thyroid hormone is also indirectly involved in sex hormone production, insulin metabolism, and growth hormone. Copper is required for the utilization of iodine, so it's possible to experience thyroid disturbances even when you are consuming adequate iodine. Symptoms of hypothyroidism include fatigue, low sex drive, weight gain, hair loss, depression, constipation, dry skin and hair, and goiter. Symptoms of hyperthyroidism include excessive sweating, weight loss, irritability, frequent bowel movements, bug eyes, and goiter.

K - Potassium interacts with sodium and chloride in the conduction of nerve impulses as well as many other functions. The average potassium intake in America has fallen below the recommended level, and all the sodium added during food processing makes the deficiency worse. Potassium is easily absorbed and there is essentially no storage in the body so make sure you get enough everyday. Symptoms of potassium deficiency are muscle weakness and mental apathy.

Li - **Lithium** is a trace mineral that has been used successfully to treat depression. Early onset of depression is a worldwide phenomenon happening at younger and younger ages. Today, one in four women and one in ten men will develop depression, mostly caused by a lithium deficiency and high sugar consumption. Other symptoms of lithium deficiency are manic depression, hyperactivity, and ADD.

Mg - **Magnesium** is essential for using carbohydrates for energy, nerve conduction, muscle contraction, protein synthesis, more than 300 enzymes, and is part of your bones.

Over 80% of magnesium is lost from grains when the outer layers are removed to make white and enriched flour. Some signs of magnesium deficiency include neuromuscular problems, depression, weakness, asthma, soft tissue calcification, tremors, and many others. *Excess magnesium can inhibit bone calcification, and excess calcium can induce signs of magnesium deficiency.*

Mn - **Manganese** is essential for glucose metabolism, energy production, bone formation, and the production of superoxide dismutase your body's internal anti-oxidant. Manganese also is involved in several enzyme systems, the development of the inner ear bones, and joint cartilage. A manganese deficiency can result in Repetitive Motion Syndrome, TMJ, and Carpal Tunnel Syndrome. These ailments cost American businesses over 20 billion dollars a year. Other symptoms of manganese deficiency include chondromalcia, asthma, loss of libido, poor cartilage formation, and retarded growth rate.

Mo - Molybdenum forms part of three essential enzymes. The average American daily intake is 75-110 mg per day. The recommended daily requirement (RDA) is 250 mg. Too much molybdenum interferes with copper metabolism.

N - Nitrogen is the structural atom in protein, DNA, and other organic molecules. The availability and usability of nitrogen from foods can vary. Nitrogen balance is a test used to determine protein uptake. A positive nitrogen balance means that your body is getting enough protein from the diet. A negative nitrogen balance means that your body is breaking down muscles and other protein structures to provide for inadequate protein consumption in you diet.

Na - Sodium is intimately associated with potassium (K) and chloride (Cl) to maintain normal water balance, normal muscle irritability, and normal acid-base balance in the body. The value of salt (NaCI) dates back to ancient times. Little or no salt is found in grains, fruits or vegetables so vegetarians require larger qualities. So much sodium is added to our food that most people would benefit from using a salt substitute that is high in potassium.

Ni - Nickel functions as a co-factor in enzymes, and facilitates the absorption of iron and zinc. Vitamin B12 is necessary for the optimal biological function of nickel. Symptoms of nickel deficiency include poor growth, dermatitis, and lowered zinc absorption.

O - Oxygen is the most critical element required for human life. Without it we can only survive for about four minutes. We get oxygen in the air we breathe, and it is the structural atom in water (H20). There is concern over the declining amount of oxygen found in our atmosphere. According to estimates, our atmosphere contained 38 percent oxygen as little as 100 years ago. During the industrial revolution that amount has dropped to 21 percent and is only 19 percent today. Most disease causing organisms (viruses and bacteria) flourish better in low oxygen environments. At the same time, low oxygen environments weaken our cells.

P - Phosphorus is an extremely important essential mineral. It is a major structural mineral for bones and teeth. Phosphorus is involved in the ATP energy cycle of every cell, and in red blood cell metabolism, as well as a multitude of other functions. Phosphorus is everywhere in food, especially in proteins. A lot of phosphorus is added in food processing so deficiency is rare. Instead, excess phosphorus (processed foods, and soft drinks) increases your calcium requirements. Most Americans are overloaded with phosphorus, aggravating osteoporosis, arthritis, high blood pressure, and other symptoms associated with calcium deficiency.

Pb - Lead has long been known to be toxic above certain blood levels. Children with mineral deficiencies often develop cravings for non-food items such as paint, dirt, sand, and are especially susceptible to lead poisoning. Lead poisoning is treated with calcium and other minerals.

S - Sulfur is an atom found in most proteins from sulfur containing amino acids (cystine, cysteine, and methionone). Glutathione is one of the strongest anti-oxidants in your body and is made from the sulfur containing amino acid cysteine. Studies have shown that whey protein can enhance your immunity by up to 500 %, one reason maybe that whey protein has a much higher cysteine level than other proteins. Symptoms of sulfur deficiency include degenerative types of arthritis involving cartilage, ligaments, and tendons, as well as other collagen diseases.

Se - Selenium is an efficient anti-oxidant and is found in enzyme systems with glutathione. One of selenium's many anti-oxidant properties is protecting lipids (fats) from peroxidation (going rancid inside the body). High intake of vegetable oils plus a selenium deficiency is the fast track to a heart attack. Selenium deficiency in adults is associated with heart disease, age spots, chronic fatigue syndrome, lowered immunity, muscle soreness, multiple sclerosis, Alzheimer's Disease, ALS, cirrhosis of the liver, pancreatitis, cataracts, and cancer. There is evidence that selenium may significantly delay the onset of full blown AIDS in HIV infected individuals. Selenium can be very toxic in excess of 800 mcg per day and, as with all nutrients, should not be used alone.

Si - Silica is essential for normal bone growth. Silica supplementation can increase the collagen in growing bone by 100 percent. Silica deficiency is characterized by dry brittle hair, brittle finger and toe nails, poor skin quality, and arterial disease.

V - Vanadium is essential for normal growth and seems to function in a way similar to insulin by altering cell transport. Vanadium may also enhance insulin's effect by making cell membrane insulin receptors more sensitive. Therefore vanadium is especially beneficial to people with glucose tolerance problems, like hypoglycemia, insulinemia, and diabetes. Vanadium can also be toxic and is required only in minute amounts. Symptoms associated with vanadium deficiency are slow growth, obesity, cardiovascular disease, diabetes, hypoglycemia, and high cholesterol.

Zn - Zinc is essential to more than 70 enzymes and is required for growth, the immune system, testosterone production, sperm formation, and sexuality. Excess zinc interferes with copper and iron metabolism and vise-versa. Never take minerals singularly! Zinc deficiency is common and may be partially responsible for the high incidence of impotence in American men. Other symptoms of zinc deficiency are pica (wool or hair eating), decrease sense of taste and smell, lowered immunity, inhibited growth, hair loss, depression, prostate enlargement, and many degenerative diseases.

ABOUT THE AUTHOR

Dr. Shannon Alexander attended Arizona State University and Western States Chiropractic College and has been a practicing chiropractor since 1988. As he began to facilitate the healing of his patients' bodies, he noticed striking similarities in those patients who had chronic conditions. This lead to years of study that uncovered the underestimated role that nutrition played in the health of his patients.

Over the next fourteen years, Dr. Alexander found that virtually everyone lacked a nutritional plan that was complete enough to be effective. In an effort to establish an all- inclusive nutritional base he developed Nutrall, a state of the art, nutrient-dense meal replacement that provides over 60 essential nutrients. The Nutrall program has been refined over the last seven years, and Dr. Alexander wanted to share his wealth of knowledge about nutrition. He wrote *The Eating Game* to give clear, concise scientific information on our modern food supply, the truth about weight loss, and a method to simplify good nutrition.

The program has also proven helpful for chronic diseases such as multiple sclerosis, arthritis, Crohn's disease, and others. It has also helped to ease the discomfort of chemotherapy.

Dr. Alexander also has done post-graduate training in acupuncture and personal training. He is an expert freestyle skier, races motocross and has a black belt in martial arts. He resides in Seattle, Washington.